Llewellyn's

Herbal
Almanac
2001

Editing/design: Michael Fallon
Interior Art: Mary Azarian
Cover Design: Lisa Novak

ISBN 1-56718-966-0
Llewellyn Publications
P.O. Box 64383 Dept.966-0
St. Paul, MN 55164

Table of Contents

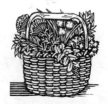

Growing and Gathering Herbs

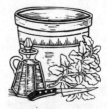

Culinary Herbs

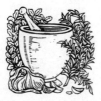

Herbs for Health

Herbs for Beauty

Herb Crafts

Herb History, Myth, and Magic

Growing
and
Gathering
Herbs

Troubleshooting the Herb Garden

By Penny Kelly

*A*lthough nothing seems to grow as willingly and trouble-free as an herb, if one of your beloved plants is not doing well, it may be worth the effort in the long run to find out why—even though this process can be an involved one.

Sun and Soil

To start, the first set of questions have to do with where the herb is planted. Is the plant in the Sun and prefers some shade? Or is the opposite true. Many herbs do just fine in full Sun, but some do better with sun only in the morning and shade in the afternoon. Such plants include caraway, chamomile, chervil, coriander, lemon balm, pennyroyal, summer savory, and valerian. On the other hand, if yarrow is in the shade it will become stringy, weak, and less resilient. Consider moving it to full sun for better health.

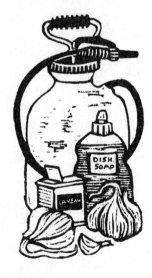

If the sun is not the problem, the next thing to check the soil. Quite a few people start out thinking that plants will always do better if the soil is top quality, enriched with compost or fertilizer, and well-watered. While this may be true for vegetables and flowers, you cannot generalize with herbs. Many herbs thrive in relatively dry, waste-soil areas, and some even prefer to restore poor or disturbed soils. Some herbs, such as red clover or burdock, do an excellent job of breaking up heavy clays or hardpan. Others, such as stinging nettles, can take poor, stony dirt and turn it into a rich loamy soil. In fact, many herbs don't do as well in rich, moist soil as they do in soils that are thin, sandy or gravelly, and found in out-of-the way places. This is because they can grow too rapidly in rich soil, and end up sprawling like drunken sailors—stems stringy and lacking in strength, leaves small and widely spaced, flavor bland because the plant has concentrated on structural growth instead of producing its essential oils. Herbs that seem to lose flavor, aroma, and oils in moist, too-rich soil are catnip, hyssop, oregano, marjoram, and sometimes lavender and thyme.

Several herbs, like rue and horehound, do better in downright poor soil with little cultivation or care, but the majority are commoners and do well in average-to-fair soil. These include the catnip, hyssop, oregano, marjoram, lavender and thyme as mentioned above, as well as bee balm, borage, calendula, caraway, chamomile, chervil, coriander, common fennel, garlic, nettles, rosemary, sage, St. John's wort, summer and winter savory, tarragon, valerian, and yarrow.

At the same time, there are some herbs that prefer the deeply-dug, rich-with-humus, well-fertilized, moist bed of soil. Basil, bay, chives, dill, Finocchio fennel, horseradish, lemon balm, spearmint, peppermint, parsley, and pennyroyal will all thrive in such a soil.

Herbs that thrive in a rich, moist, well-drained

Basil, bay leaf, chives, dill, Finocchio fennel, horseradish, lemon balm, spearmint, peppermint, parsley, pennyroyal

Herbs that thrive in poor, sandy or stony soil

Bee balm, borage, calendula, caraway, chamomile, catnip, chervil, coriander, common fennel, garlic, hyssop, lavender, marjoram, nettles, oregano, rosemary, sage, St. John's wort, summer savory, winter savory, tarragon, thyme, valerian, yarrow

Herbs that thrive in full sun

Rue, horehound

Herbs that thrive in partial shade

Basil, bay leaf, borage, calendula, catnip, chives, dill, fennel ñ both common and Finocchio, garlic, horehound, horseradish, hyssop, lavender, marjoram, the mints, nettles, oregano, parsley, rosemary, rue, sage, summer & winter savory, St. John's wort, tarragon, thyme, yarrow Bee balm, caraway, chamomile, chervil, coriander, lemon balm, pennyroyal, valerian

Watering Your Herbs

If sun and soil are not the problem, you might pay attention to how much water your herb garden is getting. In most cases, less is better. The old rule, "the garden should never go to sleep with wet feet," is doubly important in herb beds. Nothing will bring on a case of downy mildew or rot quicker than too much water, watering at the wrong time of day, or using a sprinkler head that produces big, heavy, pounding drops on your herb leaves.

Optimally, watering should be done in the earliest part of the morning—before 9 a.m. Water until the ground is saturated enough to allow little puddles to stand here and there for at least ten seconds. If you've been watering regularly, it should only take a few minutes, but if there has been a prolonged drought, your herbs may need a longer drink in order to get moisture to the deeper roots. I use a soaker hose in my herb garden, which emits a fine spray mist about three feet into the air. Once a week I turn it on in the early morning for about two hours to give the leaves a drink, then turn it over so it soaks the ground. I move it every two hours through the entire herb garden.

If you use a hose with a heavy stream of water and spray the herb leaves directly, the pressure of the water hitting the leaves can burst surface cells and cause oils to leak out of the plant. On the other hand, when the leaf is dry, the sun will cause the oil to turn black, mottled, less potent. You can still harvest and use them without harm, but the quality is not as high.

If you have had tons of rain and notice what appears to be a coating of white powder on your herb leaves, you have mildew. If this is the case, do not use chemical fungicides. These chemicals are not always able to save your crop, yet they definitely destroy the security of knowing you have poison-free herbs in your cupboard later. Most commerical fungicides are made using a combination of heavy-metal salts and estrogen-like chemicals. In your body, the metal salts damage to your blood's ability to carry oxygen and your immune system's ability to conquer infection. The estrogen-like chemicals, meanwhile, work like hormones and trigger all sorts of cell growth that is useless, or in the case of cancers, outright destructive.

Sometimes I start treatment for fungus using a light, dry dusting of Montmorillonite (also known as Bentonite) clay both on the leaves and around the base of the plant. This seems to help thwart fungus growth, and at the same time it offers a wide array of minerals to the plant. All plants are healthiest and have the best structure and nutrient content when they are in contact with a full complement of minerals; fungus indicates that the plant structure is weak and needs mineral reinforcements. If the season has been dry and you still end up with mildews or other forms of fungus, you probably need to add rock dust or paramagnetic rock powder to your soil. Add it immediately if you have it on hand, and if not, try to come up with it before the next growing season. Advertisements for paramagnetic rock and other rock dusts are often found in "Acres U.S.A.," an excellent monthly newspaper for organic growers all over the country .

While the Montmorillonite clay is working, I make a strong decoction of one or two handfuls of horsetail tea in one gallon of water. I spray this directly onto the plants, the undersides of the leaves, and the soil around the base of the plant. When I'm finished spraying, if I haven't used all the tea, I pour it into an empty gallon jug, label it, date it, and use it later. It will usually ferment in the jug and be even more powerful later on.

A spray of manure tea once a month also helps keep fungus problems from appearing. Almost any kind of manure, fresh or dried, works—cow, horse, sheep, goat, pig, chicken, rabbit, or pet dog. Though cat manure should be avoided, as it often has too many parasites in it and needs composting first. To do this, fill a large pail with about two gallons of water, then add two cups of whatever manure you have on hand. Stir the mixture well, and let it sit. The manure tea will be ready to use in a few days or a week when all the manure has sunk to the bottom of the pail. Water your herbs with this mixture in the early morning, and you will almost never be bothered by fungus diseases.

Insects

Flying, crawling, chewing insects are about the only other problem you will encounter in your herb garden, but the problems are usually minimal. Some exceptions I have encountered are leaf hoppers and aphids in dry years, Japanese beetles in the basil, and the brilliant green and black worm that feasts on parsley. The solution to the leaf hoppers and aphids has usually been a good, regular watering program, that extends into patches of ground away from the herb bed in order to lure the pests away. When all else fails, I spray with garlic tea.

This tea can be made by putting a half dozen cloves of garlic into a blender, adding a cup of water, blending vigorously to make a thin gruel, then adding four more cups of water and blending well. Pour this into a half-gallon jar to sit for three days, then strain out the garlic, add a tablespoon of anti-bacterial liquid dishsoap to the water, a tablespoon of cayenne pepper, and shake well. Put into your sprayer, add another quart of water, shake, and spray your plants with a light misting.

The garlic spray works in three ways. First, the odor of garlic offends many insects so they avoid coming around to check on what's available to eat. Second, the leafhopper, aphid, and many other insects are soft-bodied insects. When sprayed with this concoction, their bodies will dry out—bringing either complete demise or a serious inability to continue feeding. Finally, the cayenne pepper is hot enough to make chewing through the leaf an unpleasant experience for any insect. In this case, the insects aren't killed, but they are slowed down considerably.

Before taking action on any insect, though, you must ask yourself how much damage is likely to be done before harvest. Many insects can be thwarted by harvesting a bit earlier than usual. You can also plan to grow more than you need so that there is enough to feed both yourself and the insects. In fact, if you are in the habit of planting enough to share with family, friends, local critters, and insects, you can consider yourself thoughtful, less vicious, panicky, and less likely to turn to poisons when something appears to go wrong. Remember, any wise gardener knows there is always at least some level of crop damage or loss. Never fool yourself into thinking you can completely control what happens in even a tiny area or patch of ground. All you need is enough; you don't need to make a killing.

Japanese beetles are not much affected by the above spray because their hard outer shell can resist its effects. The real source of the problem with Japanese beetles is usually the gardener. When the beetles appear on your basil, it is usually because it is past time to harvest the herb. When the plant is ready to begin flowering it puts out an absolutely delicious smell that attracts the beetles. The best solution is to brush the beetles aside and begin the basil harvest immediately, before the beetles take more than their share.

In fact, my experience is that when a problem appears in the herb patch, most of the time it is due to delayed harvest. The leaves reach a peak of flavor, then as soon as the plant changes gear to flower production, the leaves begin to falter. They are less brilliant in color, less succulent, have less oil, and quickly look like they are suffering from some kind of deficiency or disease. Pick them at their peak and you'll have few problems.

As for parsley, however, this is one plant that actually does need to be watched carefully. Never assume that because a plant ordinarily does well it will do so every year. I never had problems with my parsley and never gave the plant much thought until one recent year, in late July, it struck me that the plants seemed too small for that point in the growing season. When I bent down to examine them more closely, I noticed green and black and white caterpillars munching their way along the stalks in the very center of the plants. I was horrified to see that they particularly liked the youngest, most tender shoots that were just unfurling from the plant's middle, and that was why the parsley seemed smaller and less dense than usual. Indignant at their presence, I quickly picked them off and squished them on the ground, but for over a week it was a contest to see who would have the upper hand, me or the beautiful worms. Eventually, the waves of them subsided. Later, I learned these gorgeous worms were the precursors of Monarch butterflies, and now it worries me that I haven't seen as many since.

If you have never planted an herb garden before and would like to try, keep in mind that success is really quite easy compared to other crops, and that most herbs grow well in the wild—so there is no reason to think that they would not do just as well in your garden or back yard. Many herbs are home to beneficial insects, or put out oils and scents that deter insect pests in the vegetable garden. Consider putting a couple beds of permanent herbs along each side and right down the center of your vegetable garden, any you may discover that herbs make great companions for your vegetables and as a result, less work for you.

Growing Herbs from Seed

By Penny Kelly

The first time I stepped into a commercial greenhouse, it was almost more wonderful that I could have ever imagined. Bright blooms of every color stretched before me, baskets of brilliant flowers hung overhead, and the scent of herbs wafted in the air. I had come looking for a better selection of herbs than that offered by my local hardware store, but this was beyond all expectations. An hour after I arrived, I walked out with an assortment of herbs in flats and flower pots, and a wallet that was $150 lighter. And though I'll forever recall the sensations I felt at the greenhouse, I decided the following year, in an effort to save money, that I would try growing a few of these herbs from seed.

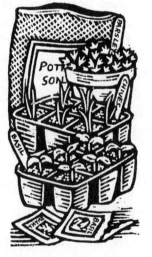

Planting Culinary Herbs

Although many people buy young herb plants from nurseries each spring, they can be grown from seed. All you need is a good information source and a lot of patience. To start, I bought my first packets of herb seed from "Seeds of Change" and "Johnny's Seeds"—two organic seed companies—since seeds produced on non-organic plants must contend with chemicals such as weed killers, pest sprays, and fungicides, and they can have problems germinating or producing strong seedlings.

When the seeds arrived I stacked them up and savored thoughts of the herb garden I would have that year. Among the varieties I had chosen were: sweet basil, lemon basil, cinnamon basil, Thai basil, holy basil, borage, calendula, caraway, chervil, regular chives, garlic chives, cilantro, dill, fennel, marjoram, nasturtium, Greek oregano, white oregano, curly parsley, Italian parsley, rosemary, summer savory, bergamot, blessed thistle, burdock, catnip, chamomile, dandelion, echinacea, elecampane, feverfew, foxglove, horehound, hyssop, anise hyssop, lady'smantle, lavender, lemon balm, licorice, marshmallow, milk thistle, milk vetch (or astragalus), motherwort, mugwort, mullein, and valerian. That I was ambitious on the first try was an understatement, yet despite my inevitable frustrations I learned a lot.

I decided back then to start my garden with the two culinary herbs that anchor much of my cooking—that is, parsley and basil. For some reason I thought parsley would be easy and basil would be difficult, so I planted an entire flat of each kind of basil with two seeds in each cell, and just a couple dozen parsley seeds. As it turned out, the reverse was true. In less than a week, I had five flats of basil, each holding well over 48 plants, but there was not a bit of parsley. I planted more parsley, watered carefully, and watched again for ten days, still with no results. I planted a third batch of seeds, watered and watched, and finally noticed the first batch was beginning to poke a tiny green leaf here and there above the soil. The basil had about an 85 percent germination rate, the parsley was slightly less than 50, and in my eagerness I had far too many of both to fit them all into the garden that year.

The directions for borage and nasturtium were to direct seed because they don't like to be transplanted, and I followed these directions with some of the seed, and then seeded a few cells to see what happened when they were transplanted. The borage did well in both cases, and within a few weeks of transplanting, you could not tell much difference between the two batches. I put them along the strawberry patch where they grew beautifully and produced dozens upon dozens of bright blue flowers that were both pretty and tasty. Oddly, the direct-seeded nasturtium failed to come up at all, while the greenhouse seedlings did just fine. They too produced masses of flowers in brilliant yellows, oranges, and reds.

The calendula and caraway were both direct-seeded as suggested. The calendula came up in about a week, while the caraway took about two weeks. The germination rate for each was 50 percent (the calendula was supposed to do much better). They grew well in the vegetable garden next to the peas, but I noticed that the part of the calendula row that was shaded for a short time of the day by the peas produced more and better looking flowers.

Chervil was sown into a flat in the greenhouse and came up well enough without a lot of fuss. When it went into the garden in rows with the other vegetables, it seemed to struggle and came up smaller than expected. I dug it up one late July evening and moved it to a flower garden in the shade of some tall pine trees where it received only a few hours of morning sun. Once it got over the shock of the transplant, it thrived.

The package of regular chives said to start them indoors, and the package of garlic chives recommended direct seeding outdoors after all chance of frost had passed. I decided to seed them both into flats in the greenhouse, and they seemed to do fine. The only problem, however, was that the markers got mixed up and I had a hard time telling which was which because the garlic chives did not smell or taste as garlicky as I thought they would.

Some dill was seeded into flats in the greenhouse, and some was direct-seeded according to the directions. It came up without a problem in both places, transplanted well, and produced generously. In contrast, the cilantro failed to come up at all.

The marjoram, oregano, and the summer savory were planted in flats in the greenhouse, and the first two seedings did not germinate. The packages instructed me to plant the seeds by pressing them lightly into the soil because they needed sunlight in order to germinate. I had never heard of such a thing before, so I covered them as usual. Of course, when nothing happened, I planted again and pressed them into soil as directed, but they kept drying out and nothing happened. In the third attempt, I put a cover of saran wrap over the flat to keep them from drying out and finally got about eight marjoram, five oregano, and ten summer savory seeds to germinate. They transplanted well, and I was glad I was persistent though I'd hoped for more plants.

Nothing I tried would induce the rosemary to germinate and grow, and finally I gave up in defeat and trotted off to the garden center to buy a few plants that someone else had started. The package of fennel seeds was overlooked completely and not planted till the next year when even two-year old seeds germinated fairly well, a little less than 50%, and grew to about 4 inches.

Medicinal Herbs

In the medicinal herb department, I was less successful, but not in ways you might expect. The bergamot, blessed thistle, milk thistle, and dandelion went into seed trays and came up easily, but once I saw that the two types of thistle actually looked like thistles, I chickened out at planting time, unable to get myself to plant something that I had always considered a weed and which regularly invaded my yard and garden. Ditto for the dandelion. The bergamot, meanwhile, transplanted well, but after the first year I discovered how invasive it was and have been struggling to keep it in check ever since.

The burdock was planted in a flat in the greenhouse but should have been direct-seeded into the garden as its tap root grows too quickly for greenhouse sowing. After the burdock sat too long in the trays, I planted about six of the best looking ones in the garden, but they were stunted for life.

With quite of few of the herbs I had moderate, sometimes disturbing, success. I direct-seeded the catnip and lemon balm, and both came up quickly. I realized later that I should have seeded the catnip into a flat in the greenhouse and then transplanted just what I needed, as it spread everywhere. The lemon balm, too, was almost as bad in its tendency to pop up everywhere.

The chamomile, elecampane, and feverfew needed light to germinate and reacted similar to the marjoram above. Once transplanted, however, they were worth the effort. The chamomile grew abundantly, the elecampane was at least six feet tall and very stately, and the feverfew was pretty and useful.

Both kinds of hyssop went into a flat in the greenhouse and after transplanting, developed into beautiful, evergreen-like plants that are both decorative and useful. I decided that I loved hyssop, even though I did not know what to do with it until I discovered how it can clear lungs and sinuses when used in a steamer.

I planted about six cells of horehound, and only two came up, but they transplanted well. That winter I made a tea of it when I caught a cold, and discovered how ungodly bitter it was. The marshmallow and mullein were both direct-seeded and didn't come up as plentifully as I'd hoped, but they did well enough to establish a small bed of each. The valerian package indicated that the seeds needed to be stratified (pre-chilled) so I put the unopened package of seeds into the freezer and left them there for a week. I planted them in a flat in the greenhouse where only about 30% of them came up, just enough to make a small bed.

The motherwort and mugwort came up quickly and without difficulty via direct seeding, and then, to my great frustration, they became "weeds" in both vegetable and flower gardens that I did battle with for years. I decided to abandon the attempt to grow them in the garden and instead to pick only wild plants.

Sparkling Successes

Among my most sparkling successes were the foxglove and lavender. I didn't know what to expect and was delighted when almost all of these came up—the foxglove having been seeded in four flats, quite slow coming up, and nearly microscopic at first. In the end it grew and transplanted well and formed a breathlessly beautiful background for the entire herb garden the next year. The lavender did almost as well. I seeded it into a flat in the greenhouse, watered it, and it gave me about twenty-five plants out of the forty-eight planted. They transplanted into several areas of the garden and flourished without fuss.

The echinacea angustifolia was successful, although somewhat accidentally. For some reason, I never read the back of the package and just put the seeds into the flat and expected them to grow. When they didn't come up, I became frustrated and only then discovered that echinacea needed to be stratified, much like valerian, so I put the seed in the freezer and took it out a week later to plant. Still, nothing happened. By May, it rather late in the season for starting anything, but I went scouring for more information and discovered in one of my references the advice to let the moist seed stratify in a refrigerator, not the freezer, for up to twelve weeks. Determined to get some echinacea from seed and thus avoid buying a pot containing a single plant for a hefty five dollars, I got out a small, square Rubbermaid container used to hold leftovers from dinner. In the bottom of it I put a wet paper towel on which I sprinkled the last forty-odd of the echinacea seeds, put the cover on, and put it in the refrigerator to stratify properly. Of course, I promptly forgot about these seeds, and didn't actually plant them until the following Spring, and they turned out to be quite exquisite.

Planting Failures

Among the more dismal of the failures were lady's mantle, licorice, and milk vetch. No matter what I did, I was not able to figure out what these three herbs needed. Much later, while reading more deeply about licorice, I discovered it was similar to rosemary, a tender perennial that should be harvested beginning in the second or third year. Perhaps it is just too cold in Michigan for licorice growing anyway. At the same time, the instructions for milk vetch said to "scarify" them, which indicates that the seed coat is so hard, so water resistant, that you need to put a small nick in the seed that will help the seed soak up enough water to swell into germination. I did this to no avail. I nicked them, and then soaked them to give them a head start, but nothing helped. As for milk vetch and lady's mantle, Mother Nature has kept me in the dark. I still do not know what went wrong with them or what I may need to do to get healthy plants from these seeds.

And so, thus concludes the saga of my first year of growing herbs from seeds. Not a bad haul overall, and most importantly, I had the satisfaction of knowing I was doing the job myself, learning more about the mysteries of the natural world, and gaining an appreciation of the difficult work of herbalists through the ages. I hope you will take on this satisfying task too some day.

Herbs: A Harvest of Pure Flavor

≈ By Penny Kelly ≈

Nothing enhances the taste, digestibility, or healing power of foods as herbs do. And, as far as it goes, no store-bought herb can compare to the levels of taste, flavor, color, and quality that you can grow and harvest in your own herb garden. Here are some good tips on how to grow and treat your own herbs and therefore utilize their qualities.

Like vegetables and fruits, herbs have a peak moment of color, flavor, and potency. At Lily Hill Farm, I grow about twenty culinary herbs as annual "must-haves" in the herb garden, with the goal to end up with several quart-size mason jars filled with elegantly dried leaves of each of our favorites. Most of what I have learned through the years about herbs has been through trial and error, and by studying a variety of resource books.

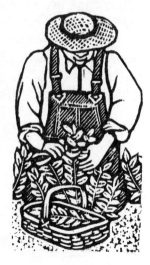

General Rules for Good Harvest Results

There are several rules of thumb to keep in mind when planning to harvest herbs for top flavor and quality. Probably the most important of these is that all herbs you harvest the leaf from reach their peak of flavor just before flowering, and those from which you harvest the flower are at their peak as soon as the flower is just open.

In general, you should gather all herbs from which you harvest the leaf after the morning dew has dried and before 10:00 am. Gather all herbs from which you harvest the flower after 10:00 am, and before the evening dew reappears—but preferably not between the hours of 11:00 am and 1:00 pm.

Furthermore, do not rinse your herbs after gathering unless they are extremely dirty or muddy. You will be more comfortable not rinsing if you do not spray your herb plants with chemical fertilizers, pesticides, herbicides, or fungicides. Such chemical fertilizers may make your herbs big but they will have weak plant structure with swollen, watery leaves that are prone to mildew and insect attack. Remember, the biggest plant is not always the best in quality. Use manure teas or compost for healthy plants.

The night before you intend to harvest, water your herbs lightly from overhead sprinklers to remove dust and dirt. The next morning, as soon as the leaves are dry, gather what you need using scissors or plant shears to carefully cut stems here. Try not to bruise the leaves when handling them, for this causes the leaves' essential oils to come to the surface of the leaves, turning it black. Basil needs an especially gentle hand.

Drying Herb Leaves

Herbs can be dried in several ways, and I have tried them all. Herbs should never be dried at temperatures higher than 115 degrees. The whole object of growing and drying your own herbs is to preserve their essential oils, enzymes, and as many of the vitamins and minerals as possible. At higher temperatures, oils evaporate, enzymes begin dying, and vitamins and minerals dissipate. Without question the best results are gained with a good dehydrator. Air drying on screens is an option, though a good indoor space is preferable for this. When I once tried to dry herbs on screens under a shady tree, the leaves lost color, some kind of sticky substance from the tree ended up all over the herb leaves, the leaves blew away in the wind, and leaves grew mildew during a humid spell. If you have a bit of time, you can also hang herbs to dry in small bunches in ventilated and darkened rooms. Direct sunlight will react with the leaves and make them rancid. As soon as the leaves are dry, put them away in an airtight container, or they will lose color, oils, flavor, and taste.

For a while I dried herbs in the microwave and thought I had found the perfect solution to the drying problem. It was quick and easy, and resulted in beautiful color and flavor in the leaves. Unfortunately, I later discovered that the heat of the microwave likely caused the essential oils of the leaves to undergo chemical changes. Not only might the oils then be unusable by human boides, they could actually become toxic.

When our application for organic certification indicated that foods or plants of any kind that were processed with microwaves could not be included in organic certification, I dropped that method and bought an Excalibur dehydrator. The results have been better than I had even dreamed. Leaves dried in this device retain their bright color and strong flavor.

When my herbs come out of the dehydrator, off the screens, or off the small clothesline in my pantry, a small bit of processing must be done. Leaves must be taken off the stems. The stems then go into the compost, and the crushed leaves are gently placed into a quart mason jar and stored using air-tight mason jar lids and bands, out of the light and away from heat and moths. They will stay colorful and flavorful for a year.

Guidelines for Specific Herbs

The first herbal references I read had little information about herb harvesting. Below are some tips I have learned since then.

Basil—Cut individual basil stems with scizzors after the plant is a foot high, and before it flowers, when the basil leaves are well-shaped. At their peak, basil leaves give off a sweet odor before the flowers appear. Once the flowers appear, flavor drops as the plant pours all its energy into the making of flowers and seeds. The smell also attracts bees and insects such as Japanese beetles.

Borage and chamomile—You are harvesting flowers here, not leaves, and with both herbs you want to select those flowers that are just open. It is hard to go wrong with these two herbs, but keep in mind that when the flower is at perfect flavor and quality for you, it is also at perfect flavor and quality for bees. When the bees stop competing with you, the flower isn't worth picking any more. Use fresh borage flowers in your salads, and use fresh or dried chamomile flowers to make teas.

Caraway—Caraway is a feathery looking plant, about two or three inches in height, that puts out a flat white flower. What you want to harvest with caraway is the seed. Once the flower has been pollinated, seeds will grow where each tiny flower was, at first green in color, but soon turning brown. To harvest, take a bowl out to the patch every other day and lean the flower head over the edge of the bowl. Lightly tap the stem against the bowl to collect the seeds that are ready to fall off. Let the seeds dry in an open container so they don't mildew once you put them in a tightly covered jar.

Chevril—Sometimes called "gourmet parsley," chervil is easy to harvest at peak. Watch for the first buds of the plant's white flowers to begin forming, then immediately cut the leaves, and use them. Drying chevril leaves diminishes the plant's qualities somewhat. You can sometimes get several cuttings from chervil if you judiciously cut only the stems that are beginning to form flower buds.

Chives—A common favorite, this ancient, onion-flavored herb should be cut about two or three inches above the plant base once it has become established and before flower stalks start to form. This is another herb that loses something in the drying process.

Coriander—This always seems to me to be a fussy plant with a stringy habit and small amount of reward at harvest time. Once coriander puts out flowers and the flowers are pollinated, the green and perfectly round seeds make an excellent harbest. I like to leave them on the plant for as long as possible to improve their flavor. I dry them in the dehydrator right on the stems, remove the seeds by hand once they're dry, and store them in pint mason jars.

Dill—This tall, marvelous plant can be harvested for its leaves, seeds, or flowers. If you want the leaves, cut the entire plant just before it flowers, then dry in the dehydrator. If you want the flowers, wait until they are in full bloom and cut. If you want the seed, wait until the flower has been pollinated and gone to seed. When the tips of the seeds begin to turn brown, cut the stem under the flower head, then take inside to air dry on a large flat screen or cookie sheet or in a paper bag.

Marjoram—One of my favorite herbs, marjoram is easy to grow and harvest. Watch for signs of flowering (marjoram has an unusual, rounded green flower), then cut the entire plant off just above the ground so as not to miss even one of its pungent leaves. I have found that even if it does go to flower, it retains excellent flavor and taste. If you are late with the marjoram harvest, cut and dry the entire plant, stems, leaves, flowers and all.

Oregano—Easy to grow and simple to harvest, I harvest oregano two or three times each year. To harvest, cut the stems about two inches above the base of the plant before it flowers. Oregano must be watched, like basil, because it, too, has an optimal stage of green perfection. If you don't get your oregano at this point, the flowers start blooming, the plant begins to sprawl, the stems fall to the side and try to root themselves in the soil, the leaves become mottled with black spots.

Parsley—When harvesting parsley, cut older, larger, lower, darker green stems around the edges of the plant when they get to be about six to eight inches or longer, and leave the middle of the plant alone to keep producing. If you have curly parsley, it will be very tightly curled when the leaves first emerge and by waiting until it uncurls just a little, the light striking the leaf surface will produce more clorofyll, which is good for you and flavorful. If you have the flat, Italian version, cut the thicker, longer stems first and leave the rest to grow. You do not have to worry about the plant flowering because parsley does not flower until the second year.

Rosemary—Begin harvesting rosemary when the plant is about eight inches tall. Pinch or cut off the ends of the various branches.

Savory (Summer and Winter)—The savories are quite different from one another. One is annual, one is perennial; one is leggy, the other close-growing; one lighter green, the other quite dark. But harvest is simple for both: cut individual stems before flowering, then dry, and store. Watch the plant closely, though, because the white flowers are tiny, they always seem to appear overnight, especially on summer savory, and savory is one of the plants where there is a truly noticeable drop in flavor and taste after flowering.

SAGE (Regular, Clary, Pineapple, etc.)—Sage does very well when individual stems are cut and put into small bunches to hang dry. In the summer, sage produces beautiful flowers that are very attractive to bees. When the flowers are long gone, and autumn is about to arrive, I often harvest again. The flavor seems to be even stronger in autumn sage, and the leaves bigger.

Mint (Spearmint, Peppermint, Chocolate, Lemon, Apple, Catnip)—I collect spearmint early in the spring because I like the milder flavor. By the time the plant is two feet tall and ready to flower, the flavor is much stronger and suitable for medicinal purposes. For peppermint, chocolate, apple mint, and catnip I wait until just before flowering and then trim individual stems about four inches above the root base. For lemon mint, I harvest leaves until I have enough, then let the plant flower and trim off the flowers for using in potpourri or even muffins.

Tarragon—The distinctive flavor of tarragon is best captured by harvesting in the morning after the dew has dried and before the sun gets too hot. French tarragon forms graceful stems with long, narrow leaves and almost never flowers, while Russian tarragon flowers profusely, produces seed prodigiously, and will take over the garden. Watch to see which kind you have, making sure you harvest anything that looks like it's about to flower.

Thyme (Regular and Lemon)—Thyme is easy to grow and harvest. A low-growing plant with tiny leaves that produces well from spring to frost, it's best harvested for flavor before flowering. Cut new growth off about two inches above the base of the plant.

Once you get used to growing and harvesting your own herbs, you will never be satisfied with commercially produced herbs again. Not only is the flavor difference a night and day affair, there is often an unexpected connection to ancient ritual that you become unwilling to break.

A Healing Garden Layout

❧ By Elizabeth Barrette ❧

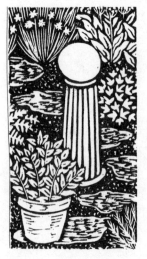

*H*erbs offer a wealth of culinary, magical, and medicinal benefits. With a careful plan, you can bring together a selection of plants prized for their healing powers. The plans described here should serve as inspiration that you can customize according to your needs.

First, you should strive to create a garden whose serene mood promotes positive emotions. To do this, a garden plan should build around an elliptical garden plot, which draws its shape from the soft curves of nature and evokes images of eggs, breasts, and sacred springs. Two curving paths can allow easy access to the middle of the garden, and provide a means to get close to your health-giving plants.

Furthermore, when selecting garden components such as statues, stepping stones, and the like, make certain you choose ones safe for outdoor use in your climate. In the variable Midwest climate, for instance, certain plants—mentioned below—tend to grow well, but if you live in an area prone to extremes of rainfall or temperatures, you may want to make a few substitutions.

Things You Will Need for the Garden

Plants—Echinacea, fennel, fenugreek, feverfew, garlic, horehound, hyssop, lavender, lemon balm, mullein, peppermint, roman chamomile, rose, rosemary, sage, thyme, vervain, wintergreen, yarrow

Objects—Medium-sized smooth river stones for edging, enough stepping stones for two paths, several bags of bark chip mulch, small accent statuettes or other decorative items, a pair of large flowerpots, a centerpiece

Healing Garden Layout

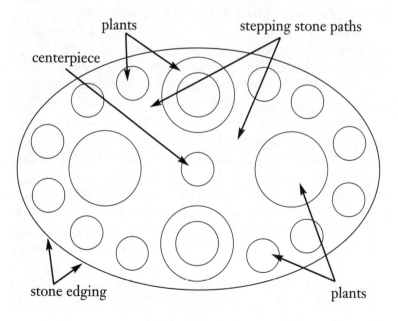

Getting Started with Plants

Depending on the size of garden you want, your plant quantities may vary a bit. If you buy seeds, you will need one packet each of fenugreek, feverfew, horehound, hyssop, lavender, lemon balm, peppermint, rosemary, sage, vervain, and yarrow; plus one or two packets each of echinacea, fennel, mullein, roman chamomile, and thyme. Many of these do come as plants at local nurseries; if you buy yours this way, consult the label for recommended spacing. Rose and wintergreen are best acquired as plants, and garlic comes in bulbs. You will need one rose, about a dozen wintergreen plants, and one bulb of garlic, which breaks down into cloves that you plant individually.

For best results, lay out the garden space before you start planting. Prepare the soil and mark boundaries. Add the stepping stones to give yourself a place to stand while working on the middle. Begin planting in the center and work your way outward. After all the planting is done, cover open soil between plantings with a layer of bark mulch to keep it from getting muddy.

Wintergreen forms a low carpet around the centerpiece, growing to six inches. The pinkish berries and leathery green leaves persist through the coldest months, giving the garden winter interest. Oil present in the plant contains methyl salicylate, a relative of aspirin that is easily absorbed through the skin. This astringent oil relieves muscle aches and rheumatism. The leaves make a tasty tea useful for treating headaches, muscle aches, and sore throats. Wintergreen's magical properties include healing, hex-breaking, and protection.

Fennel, both green and bronze varieties, grows tall at the back of the garden—up to six feet. You can chew fennel seeds to sweeten your breath, aid digestion, or assuage hunger. They also make an excellent flavoring for breads, fish, fruit pies, and other foods. Tea brewed from the seeds increases breast milk, regulates the menstrual cycle, and relieves constipation. The feathery leaves may be used fresh in seafood or salad dressings. Magically, use fennel for healing, purification, or protection.

Roman chamomile forms a low ring around the fennel; it grows up to six inches and has a similarly delicate leaf structure. This herb is most famous for yielding a soothing tea, made from dried flowers and good for treating stomach troubles or insomnia. Save the used tea bags; used as a poultice, they reduce inflammation and dark shadows under the eyes. A decoction of the flowers also brightens and conditions light-colored hair. Sprinkle chamomile around your home for prosperity and protection; it is also used in incenses for sleep or meditation.

Rose fills the center left of the garden, and you can reach it from the path running between it and the centerpiece. Choose a vigorous, fragrant variety known for producing plenty of rose hips; these usually grow about five feet high. A peaceful color such as pink or white will suit a healing garden better than hot shades of red, yellow, or orange. Rose-flower water revives dry, tired skin; it also adds exquisite flavor to desserts and beverages. (Try adding a dash to strawberry milkshakes.) Process rose hips into tea, wine, jelly, or syrup. All rose hips contain vitamin C, but several cultivars offer extraordinary amounts. Tea brewed from the leaves has a mild laxative effect. Most famous for its use in love spells, rose also brings luck and promotes psychic powers.

Echinacea provides a patch of bright color at the front of the garden, growing to three feet. The pinkish-purple flowers attract butterflies, but it is the rhizome that provides the healing benefits by activating the body's immune system. Echinacea also has some antibiotic and antiviral properties. Native Americans sometimes offered this herb to the spirits to help strengthen spells.

Thyme forms a low-growing ring around the echinacea, up to six inches tall. All varieties aid the digestion of fatty foods and are used to flavor stews, meats, and fresh fruit dishes. Antiseptic oil from the leaves and flowers treats depression, respiratory complaints, and muscle aches. Wild creeping thyme also has sedative properties; it makes an excellent tea for hangovers, coughs, and sore throats. Use thyme honey to sweeten herb teas. Carrying this herb grants courage and enhances psychic powers.

Mullein fills the middle right of the garden, convenient to the path running between it and the centerpiece; this herb grows about four to five feet. Its yellow flowers lighten fair hair, reduce inflammation, and add flavor to liqueurs. The leaves and flowers also have soothing, expectorant, and spasm-calming properties useful for treating coughs, and the root serves as a diuretic. Magically, mullein guards against evil spirits and nightmares.

On the left side of the garden, individual clumps form an arc around the rose, beginning with fenugreek in the back. This herb grows to thirty inches and has a wide range of uses. Its pungeant seeds contain the vitamins A, B1, C, plus iron and other minerals. Ground and roasted, they flavor curries and chutneys; made into tea, they reduce fever, soothe digestion, and relieve menstrual pains. Hormone precursors in the seeds increase breastmilk, lower blood cholesterol, and raise libido. The leaves make a nice addition to salads. Magically, fenugreek attracts money.

Vervain goes between the fenugreek and rosemary, reaching about three feet in height. Pick the flowering tops for an infusion useful in treating cramps, jaundice, headaches, insomnia, and depression. The leaves and stems are used as a nerve tonic and liver stimulant. Pounded into a poultice, this herb also aids in healing skin ulcers and wounds. Its magical applications include protection, purification, peace, sleep, and general healing; it also governs the complementary realms of love and chastity.

Rosemary, next to vervain, grows to a height of three feet. Plant this tender perennial in a large, decorative pot so that you can take it indoors during winter. Use the pretty blue, white, or pink flowers fresh or sugar-glazed as a garnish. Rosemary leaves, popular in many dishes, help preserve food and make it easier to digest fats. They have antiseptic and antioxidant properties, and are often used in dandruff shampoos or conditioning rinses for dark hair. This herb is a favorite stuffing for magical puppets, an ingredient in incense, and a charm for memory enhancement.

Feverfew lies between the rosemary and horehound and reaches two feet. This plant produces pyrethrum, a natural compound that paralyzes many insect pests; steep the leaves for an excellent organic spray that is safe for use on most other plants. The leaves are a gentle sedative, also good for reducing inflammation and relaxing blood vessels. The pretty daisylike flowers make an infusion for treating arthritis and headaches. Carry feverfew to protect against accidents.

Horehound rests between feverfew and sage, growing to two feet. The wrinkled, woolly leaves add tactile attraction to the garden; use them for making cough syrups or medicinal candies for treating colds and sore throats. Horehound has antiseptic, expectorant, digestive, and laxative properties. Magically, it breaks hexes and drives out negative influences. Sage lies next to horehound, at the end of the arc, reaching two feet in height. It comes in many forms, with purple or white flowers, and green, purple, gold, or variegated leaves. This popular cooking herb adds flavor and improves digestion of fatty foods. Dry the leaves to make an antiseptic, tonic tea. Its magical powers include protection, life extension, and the granting of wishes.

On the right side of the garden, clumps of herbs form an arc around the mullein, beginning with yarrow in the back. This plant grows one to four feet and blooms in a wide range of colors; choose a medium-sized variety with flowers in soothing shades of white, creamy yellow, or pink. The feathery leaves have a sweet, strong scent that is uplifting and cheerful. Fresh leaves also stop bleeding when applied to small cuts and scrapes. The whole plant steeped in a bath reduces bruising by minimizing internal bleeding. The flowers have digestive and diuretic properties. Dry the stems for Druidic or I Ching divinations.

Lavender lies between yarrow and peppermint, growing from one to three feet depending on variety. Flowers may be purple, white, or pink, and are used to flavor vinegar, jam, cream, and even stew. Dried, the flower spikes are woven into ribbon-decked wands or added to potpourri. Use dried flowers to make tea for treating bad breath, dizziness, digestive upsets, headaches, and nervousness. Essential oil of lavender has analgesic, antiseptic, and relaxing properties. In magical use, this herb brings peace, happiness, and longevity.

Spearmint grows between lavender and lemon balm, reaching two to three feet. Plant this herb in a large pot to keep it from taking over the whole garden. It can flavor desserts, vegetables, and sauces; also, the leaves may be sugar-coated for garnishes. Spearmint tea improves digestion, minimizes flatulence, and stimulates the body. This plant also has antiparasitic, antiseptic, and sweat-inducing properties. Magically, it enhances mental powers and promotes healing.

Lemon balm lies between spearmint and hyssop, growing to a height of two feet. Use the fresh leaves in vinegars, oils, and fish recipes. They also soothe insect bites, and lemon balm tea relieves headaches and digestive upsets. The refreshing scent invigorates and banishes melancholy thoughts. Magical applications include love, success, and healing.

Hyssop fits between lemon balm and garlic, reaching two feet in height. Flowers come in blue, white, or pink. The leaves lend a sharp flavor to dishes and help digest fat. They also make a sedative, expectorant tea good for colds, flu, or bronchitis. Pounded into a poultice, the leaves soothe wounds and bruises. Hang this herb in the home to disperse evil and purify.

Garlic completes the arc next to hyssop, growing up to two feet high. Its powerful flavor enhances savory dishes. This herb lowers cholesterol and blood pressure, minimizes acne outbreaks, and purifies blood. Added to cold remedies, it clears phlegm, but usually requires another strong herb to mask the flavor. It also contains valuable vitamins and minerals, and in addition to its aphrodisiac and healing uses, garlic banishes evil.

The Objects

Smooth river stones outline this garden, keeping the mulch in place. Set these around the perimeter. You can collect your own, or purchase them from a building supply or garden center. Lay them out to form two curving paths through the center of the garden. The left path begins at the front of the garden between sage and thyme, then passes between rose and wintergreen, and ends at the back between fenugreek and Roman chamomile. The right path begins between garlic and thyme, goes between mullein and wintergreen, and ends between yarrow and Roman chamomile.

Accent statuettes and a pair of large, ornamental pots add interest. Choose small or medium figures that make you feel peaceful and serene. Set them in the open, or hide them playfully in the foliage. Select pots with suitable motifs like leaves, Celtic knotwork, and so forth. The focal point of your garden should be a find centerpiece. This can be anything that evokes the healing energies you desire. Representational statues of suitable deities include Brigid, the Venus of Willendorf, Taueret, Apollo, Bona Dea, Hotei, and Hypnos. Other likely images include children, fairies, or guardian angels, as well as serpents, bears, owls, and other animals that have been associated with healing. More abstract options include a birdbath, Celtic cross, water fountain, or Japanese stone lantern. A gazing ball is especially nice—these come in green, silver, gold, and other colors.

Enjoying Your Garden

This garden will become a special healing sanctuary for you as you make use of the herbs in magical, medicine, and food, and as other creatures—bees, toads, butterflies, and birds—move in and add life to the place. Many people find that working in a garden makes them feel calm and happy.

Perhaps you will even choose to share your garden with others. It can serve as a focus for ritual or meditation, and you may wish to dedicate this space as a shrine to the healing power of your choice. You can also use it as a teaching garden for students of herbalism or other healing disciplines. Whatever you decide, growing a garden like this offers many opportunities for unleashing the healing power of body, soul, and spirit.

Companions in the Herb Patch

≈ By Penny Kelly ≈

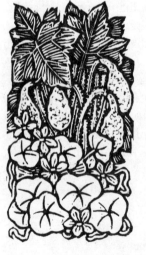

Except for the possibilities of romance, a good companion in the world of plants is not much different from a good love companion for you or me. That is to say, the right companion can make life healthier and more productive, with less stress from competition or the interfering annoyances of pests. With humans as well as with plants, there is little scientific understanding of exactly how this works; all we do know is that some plants are great company for one another.

In the lore of plants, as in the lore of love, much of what we know has been passed down from gardeners of ancient times—passed by word of mouth over the back fence, or among family members. What we do know about companion planting, also known as plant symbiosis, is that plants really do affect each other. Some effects are clearly physical, as when the presence of two plants causes both to grow better. The reasons for these effects are murky: some plants give off heat to plants around them, others provide some amount of windbreak or shade, and all plants attract and host insects that may be beneficial. Physcial factors in plants include the size and amount of space given plants will take up, whether or not they demand water and nutrients in the same time, the amount of mulch they create in dropping leaves and stems at the end of the growing season, and the chemical components in their leaves and stems.

Plants also affect each other chemically, via aroma, exudations from the leaves, and by release of humic acids from the roots. Although there seems to be little hard science in book form on the subject, an understanding of how plant oils heal humans to get a better understanding of how plants may affect one another. For instance, it is fairly common knowledge that all plants manufacture oils. Sesquiterpins, a chemical found in the oil of many herbs, have the extraordinary capacity to cross the blood-brain barrier and set up frequency resonances in the brain that directly and powerfully affect the function of the whole body-mind system. This is the basis of aromatherapy, and with this in mind, it is not too much to imagine that a local grouping of vegetables, fruits, and flowers would be affecting one another in similar ways.

The same thing happens at the root levels when roots of one plant intertwine with another. If one plant needs to dissolve a quantity of a particular mineral from the soil, it will produce certain acids which it excretes through its root hairs. The acid goes to work upon stones, soil crumbs, or whatever the source of the mineral might be, and when the mineral is freed, the plant takes it in through the process known as transpiration. In this way, plants search out and absorb whatever they need to be healthy and productive. It seems obvious that some acids released from a given plant might irritate or interfere with the activities and operations of a neighboring plant. Some plants in fact are known for their antagonism to other plants. Fennel is one of these.

Other plants are documented as beneficial companions—such as stinging nettle which increases the essential oils in neighboring herbs, and which fights aphids, black flies, and moths, and which produces a nearly perfect form of humus when its roots are allowed to rot in the ground over the fall and winter.

Even though there is not much scientific documentation to determine how companion plants help each other, there is enough anecdotal information to begin taking advantage of this phenomenon. You might want to keep some of the following traditional dos and don'ts in mind when it comes time to plant your garden next spring.

Herbs as Companions to Vegetables

Beans—Don't put garlic or nasturtiums near your green beans as they are not compatible. Do put summer savory not only in the bean patch, but in the bean pot when you cook them. Beans and savory like one another.

Beets—Beets get along with just about everyone in the herb family, especially onions. They turn their nose up at pole beans, yet don't mind bush beans or soybeans.

Brassicas—The cabbages, cauliflowers, broccolis, kohlrabis, kales, brussels sprouts, and collards of the world all have similar preferences in companions. They love dill, chamomile, sage, rosemary, wormwood, and peppermint (especially peppermint). With any of their preferred herb companions, or a bit of thyme or hyssop, you get the added benefit of keeping away the white cabbage moth. Just be sure you don't put cabbage close to the strawberries as they dislike each other immensely, and if you put the cauliflower too close to the stinging nettle, you'll get a runaway crop of nettles.

Carrots—There will be a revolt in the carrot patch if you put dill nearby. Substitute chives, lemon balm, leeks, or onion.

Corn—Almost nothing bothers corn, except perhaps fennel. Corn likes parsley and potatoes, peas and beans. Corn is a prodigious user of nitrogen, while peas and beans are prodigious suppliers of nitrogen. This makes for a nice balance of give and take among these friends.

Cucumbers—These fussy-but-delectable vegetables detest potatoes and sage, so plant them well away from each other. They like a bit of dill, but not too much.

Eggplant—No special herb companions for eggplant are known, but it does better near green beans because the green beans deter eggplant pests.

Leeks—Leeks like parsley among the herb family, and don't have many enemies. They also like celery and carrots.

Lettuces—As with cucumbers, lettuce likes a bit of dill, but not a whole row or an entire patch, just one dill here and there. Onions can be interspersed liberally with lettuce, but the best influences in producing great lettuce are strawberries and carrots.

Melons—Melons are pretty much loners and little is known about the company they prefer.

Onions—Friends of onions include chamomile and summer savory, but not en masse. A dozen feet of onion row need only one chamomile plant, and maybe two or three savory. On the vegetable side, lettuce, beets, and carrots all improve the onion crop.

Peas—Peas have lots of friends, but parsley is not among them. Neither are onions or garlic. Put these three elsewhere and your peas will thrive.

Potatoes—Put one or two nasturtiums among your potatoes, and a horseradish plant at each end of the row and you'll have healthy potatoes. This is important since potatoes are finicky. They don't do well with sunflowers, raspberries, pumpkin, cucumber, tomatoes, apple, cherry or birch wood nearby.

Pumpkins—These have no special herb friends, but they do like beans and corn, and dislike potatoes.

Radish—Putting nasturtiums among the radishes will make them tasty and flavorful, while adding some chervil will make them hot. Lettuce will make them tender, but radishes do not like hyssop at all.

Squash—Squash benefits from a few nasturtium plants among them because it helps keep the squash bugs away.

Strawberries—Borage is the best friend of strawberries and has been for many years. Spinach, lettuce, and bush beans will help if borage is not available.

Tomatoes—Tomatoes dislike dill, kohlrabi, and potatoes, but parsley is a great companion, and so are asparagus, marigolds, and stinging nettley. The marigolds influence the tomato for better growth and more fruit, while the stinging nettle gives resistance to molds and mildews.

Companions In The Herb Family

Besides helping vegetables and flowers, many herbs have favorite herbal companions and will grow better, have more flavor, and produce more oils, than when grown separately.

Anise—This tasty herb likes to be grown with coriander.

Basil—Sweet basil, like all other herbs, does better when yarrow is nearby, but will not tolerate the bitter rue at all.

Borage—This herb's only special friend is strawberries.

Caraway—Keep caraway away from fennel!

Chamomile—A little mint and a few onions are all that chamomile really needs, but be aware that the mint will suffer a bit while the chamomile flourishes.

Chevril—The radish is chervil's only special companion.

Chives—These do well alone, seldom experiencing either disease or attack from insects.

Coriander—This can keep fennel from forming seeds so keep the two apart.

Dill—This attracts bees and assists cabbages, but otherwise has no preferred companions.

Garlic—Garlic does better if roses are planted nearby, and the roses thrive as well.

Horseradish—Has no particular companions.

Hyssop—Offers friendship to grapevines, but needs no special friends to help it along.

Lavender—Although some consider lavender to be difficult to grow, my own experience is that it grows well with creeping thyme, lemon balm, pine trees, and hyssop.

Lovage—Lovage does much better close to a sage plant.

Lemon Balm—This herb is loved by many other herbs, but has no special friends of its own.

Marjoram—Like lemon balm, marjoram is friend to everyone.

Mint—If chamomile gets into the mint, you'll have poor flavor and a drop in oil production in the mint. However, stinging nettle growing close to mint will increase the oils in peppermint by over two-fold.

Nasturtums—These lovely flowering plants offer benefits to many but do not seem to need companions of their own.

Oregano—Oregano is a good companion for many herbs and vegetables. My own experience is strawberries and oregano benefit when planted next to each other.

Parsley—Both parsley and celery do better when together, but parsley seems to need no special herb companions.

Rosemary—Grows well if sage and yarrow are nearby.

Sage—A powerful aromatic that does well with rosemary.

Summer savory—If planted in cautious numbers, both summer and winter savory plants can assist onions.

Stinging nettle—This powerful herb seldom gets the praise it deserves. It helps any neighbor resist diseases, it greatly increases the amount of essential oil produced in herb plants. A patch of stinging nettles one year, followed by a cover crop of rye that overwinters before being turned under, will produce very sweet vegetables that are healthy from seedling stage to seed production stage.

Tansy—If it doesn't get away from you and take over the garden, tansy will repel all sorts of insect pests. Plant it on the west or northwest side of a garden so prevailing breezes carry its properties over the rest of the garden.

Tarragon—Loves to have a few yarrow plants nearby.

Thyme—Like tarragon, thyme is enhanced by yarrow.

Valerian—Again, yarrow is the preferred companion, as well as echinacea and foxglove.

Wormwood—The powerful chemical absinthins in wormwood make for poor companionship to almost every herb in the garden. Fennel, sage, and caraway especially.

Yarrow—This plant is everyone's friend, increasing flavor in basil, lemon balm, marjoram, mint, oregano, rosemary, sage, savory, tarragon, thyme, valerian, and wormwood.

Take some time this winter to study plant companions that seem to work well with one another, and you can begin to take advantage of plant symbiosise. You will find that gardening is easier, more pleasurable, more productive, and the vegetables, fruits, flowers and herbs are sweet and delicious. Putting your garden together this way is not only rewarding, you may find that the plants consider you to be the best companion of all.

Wild about Mint

⊰ By Carly Wall, C.A. ⊱

My relationship with herbs came suddenly. It didn't happen over months or years; I simply discovered them one day and was hooked for life—picturing the large herb garden that I would grow, imagining meandering pathways and delicious scents. When, years later I finally did have my dream garden, I mistakenly ignored warnings about planting mint. "How could anyone not have mint in their herb garden?" I asked myself.

Since then, I confess, I've cursed the day I made this decision. I'm here to warn you again: do not plant mint in your herb garden. Unless, of course, all you want is an herb garden full of mint. After all, mint spreads. Even if you plant it in a container and bury the container it spreads. It will spread even though you rip it up by the handfuls. It will spread no matter what you do and you may never be truly rid of it.

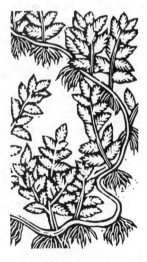

Mint, of course is a wonderful herb with many varied uses; both medicinally and culinary. But if you are going to plant it, make it an out-of-the-way place—the back of the barn, the edge of the woods, along an old fence row. And then don't worry about it—left alone, it will grow and thrive. After all these years, I no longer curse mint. Instead, I understand it. Mint just can't be contained, and it doesn't want to commune with other herbs. It merely wants to be free.

The Many Faces of Mint

In days of old, all varieties of mint were used the same way. Today we've broken down what mint is best for what usage. Peppermint, (M. piperita), is preferred in the West for medicinal usage. It's good for nausea, travel sickness, fever, and headache. It cools internally while promoting sweating, and it is good for digestion and in combatting infections. With peppermint inhalations, you can clear congestion and other bronchial problems associated with colds. Peppermint tea is good for nausea, indigestion, and gas. Pour hot water over a bunch of peppermint sprigs, wring out a cloth in this, and use as a compress for arthritic pains. Add two or three drops of peppermint essential oil to one tablespoon of water to combat ringworm or to repel mosquitoes. Or add five to ten drops in two tablespoons of almond oil as a massage oil for headaches or menstrual pain.

The nineteen pure mentha species have been cross bred intensively, and now there are more than 2000 varieties of mint. In fact, there are as many flavors of mint as you can imagine. Applemint has a fruity quality and soft gray-green leaves, and it makes a wonderful tea. Then there's something new from France called Banana mint. Chocolate mint, meanwhile, may not smell exactly like chocolate, but people say that it has a peppermint patty scent and flavor. Corsican mint is a carpet-forming mint with tiny leaves. This is great for terrariums and miniature gardens. Ginger mint has just a hint of ginger to it. Orange mint and pineapple mint have citrus-like scents that are wonderful in adding to perfumes or potpourris. And there's a strain called Kentucky Colonel Spearmint which is the best mint for making the famous Mint Julep drinks famous in Kentucky.

Then, there's the old faithful, spearmint (Mentha spicata), which is less powerful than peppermint but has about the same qualities. They say this is best for cooking—-in spicing peas, carrots, or potatoes, and in making mint jelly and mint sauces for roast lamb. You can also make distilled water with spearmint that is good for dabbing on the temples for headaches. A wash of it is good for acne and dermatitis. And spearmint is a good herb to have on hand to ease the discomforts of colds, fevers, or flu.

There are several types of spearmint—-curly (spicata var. crispa) and the aforementioned Kentucky Colonel (M. corditalia). Spearmint, probably the most popular home-grown mint, is a hardy branched perennial with bright green, lance-shaped runners and pink or lilac-coloured flowers in slender spikes. It is native to the Mediterranean area, and now common throughout Europe. When introduced into the United States, it became instantly popular as a flavoring for toothpastes, gum, and mouthwashes because of its refreshing qualities.

Growing Mint

Varieties of mint have the characteristic of having squarish stems and tooth-edged leaves. To keep plants healthy, divide or replenish your beds every four or five years to ensure healthy, vigorous growth. Mint grows best in full sun, and in well-drained soil. It is hardy to zone five. Most mint varieties produce no seed or if they do, aren't true to the parent plant because of so much hybridization. To grow a favorite strain of mint, simply propagate by using the cuttings. Mint often will in fact propagate itself so well that it can become a weed.

On problem you may encounter is a disease which can attack your mint. When it does, it is incurable and makes it necessary to destroy your plants. It is a fungus (Puccinia Mentha), called rust. It develops inside the plant and when found, you must dig up all plants that show sign of it so it will not spread. Healthy plants should be obtained, and planted far from the original spot so that the infected soil does not contaminate the new plants.

A Few Recipe Ideas

Mint Jelly—Take a recipe for making apple jelly and add some chopped mint leaves to the batch

Mint Vinegar—To make mint vinegar, merely add a handful of mint leaves to a mason jar of apple cider vinegar. Let it steep 12-14 days and strain. Mint vinegar is good as a headache remedy. Daub a cotton ball and run across the temples, or use for inhalations, or add to bathwater to cool you off on a hot day.

Mint Cake—Add chopped mint leaves to your cake mix, or add mint essential oil to your icing recipe and make a surprise mint cake. Chocolate mint cake is especially good.

Drinks—Mint is also a delight when added to drinks. Experiment with adding mint to your tea mixes, or to punch. You can also add a sprig to your glass and it is a pretty addition. Another way to add appeal is to freeze mint sprigs in flower in ice cubes and float them in your drinks.

However you use mint, it is a wonderful herb to have on hand. Just make sure it isn't inside your herb garden.

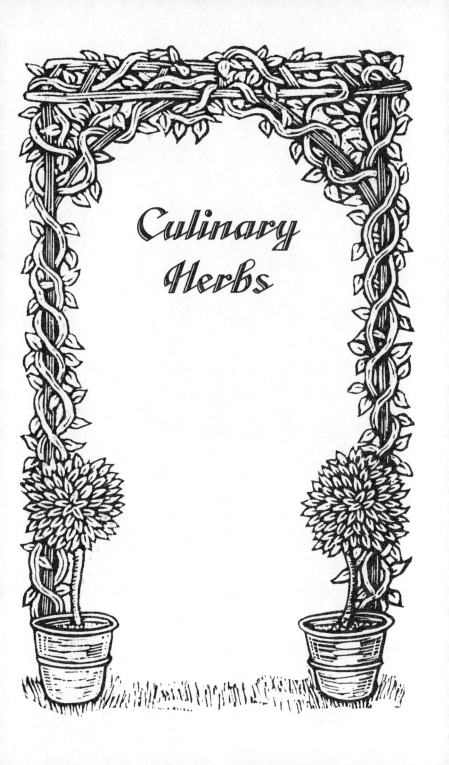

Culinary
Herbs

In the Kitchen with Lavender

≈ By Carly Wall, C.A. ≈

I will never forget my first cup of lavender tea. It was an experiment; I had just begun growing lavender and had fallen in love with it—its scent, its visual beauty, the way the plant grew, the way the bees were drawn to it, and its endless usefulness. According to the art and science of aromatherapy, I had learned, not only could lavender be used to banish headaches, but it could heal burns, repair skin wounds, and remove stress. Lavender could be used to chase away moths in a closet and repel insects in the garden. Lavender could soothe my insomniac husband, and it could gracefully decorate my home in bouquets, bundles, and potpourris.

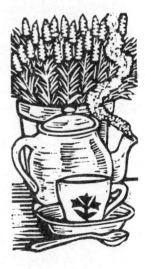

And so, when a friend and I decided to brew a cup of lavender tea, it was merely an experiment to see if indeed, lavender could be brought into the kitchen successfully. It was, of course, a complete success. The tea was delightful—sweet and flowery with a hint of a kick. We drank it with honey and enjoyed wonderful benefits—relaxation, headache relief, stress reduction. We were soon laughing and discussing the most silly subjects!

In any case, this tea was merely the beginning of my foray into lavender cooking. I've delighted in trying it in many recipes, and here I share some of my favorites. I hope this sparks a streak of experimentation for you.

Lavender Tea

To make a lavender infusion tea, add one teaspoon of lavender buds (or leaves) per each cup to a muslin bag. Fill the teapot with boiling water and add the muslin bag. Cover and let steep for five minutes. Remove the bag. Add honey to sweeten and a slice of lemon in each cup.

Lavender-Chamomile Jam

6-8 jelly jars, sterilized

2 cups apple juice

½ cup strong lavender tea

½ cup strong chamomile tea

1 cup lavender buds

1 teaspoon lemon juice

3½ cups honey

Place apple juice, teas, and lemon juice in an enamel pot. Bring to a rapid boil and leave for one minute. Add honey, lavender buds and bring back to a hard boil, leaving for two minutes or until it forms a jelled film on inserted spoon. Pour into jelly jars. Seal in a boiling water bath 15 minutes. Store in a cool place.

Lavender Sugar Cookies

½ cup fresh lavender buds

½ cup butter, room temperature

½ cup granulated sugar

1 teaspoon vanilla

pinch of salt

grated rind of 2 lemons

2 tablespoons lemon juice

2 eggs, lightly beaten

2 cups flour

2½ teaspoons baking powder

Almonds to decorate

Preheat oven to 350 degrees. Cream butter and sugar. Add lemon zest, juice, lavender, and vanilla. Beat in egg. Blend in dry ingredients. Dough will be sticky. Drop by teaspoon onto lightly sprayed cookie sheet. Top with almonds. Bake 15 minutes until light gold in color. Makes about 3 dozen cookies

Lavender Punch

6 teaspoons dried mint

6 cups boiling water

1 tablespoon dried lavender blossoms

1 liter ginger ale

1 cup purple grape juice

ice cubes with fresh mint leaf frozen in each

Infuse the mint in the water in a teapot for ten minutes. Add the lavender blossoms to the pot. Allow the tea to cool. Strain the tea and add the ginger ale, grape juice, and ice cubes. If serving in a punch bowl, float lavender buds and mint sprigs on top.

Lavender Pudding

2½ cups hot milk

¼ cup cornmeal

1 teaspoon sugar

¼ teaspoon baking soda

¼ cup fresh lavender flower buds

⅓ cup lavender syrup (See recipe below)

1 cup cold milk

½ cup raisins

Heat milk in top of a double boiler. Stir in cornmeal slowly and continue stirring until mixture thickens. Combine sugar and baking soda and stir into milk mixture. Add lavender syrup and cold milk, stir well. Add raisins. Pour into lightly oiled 1½ quart casserole dish. Bake at 275 degrees for 2 hours. Serve warm topped with vanilla ice cream.

Lavender Syrup

Crush 2 tablespoons rose hips, 1 teaspoon rose petals and 2 teaspoons lavender flowers in 2 cups boiling water. Add ¾ cup granulated sugar and stir till dissolved. Cook over low heat, stirring occasionally, till syrup is reduced and slightly thickened. Cool and strain into glass container. Store, covered, in refrigerator. Use within 2 weeks. The syrup is also good to flavor drinks, ice cream, or French toast.

Lavender Sugar

Stir together 2 cups sugar and 1 tablespoon dried lavender flowers. Store in a tightly closed container for two weeks. You may strain out the flowers or leave them in as you prefer. Use to sweeten teas or other beverages, or to sprinkle on cookies.

Lavender Vinegar

Heat a quart of apple cider vinegar to just below boiling in a nonreactive container. Remove from heat and add ½ cup dried lavender blossoms. Cover until vinegar has cooled. Pour into a large glass or ceramic container with a lid. Let infuse for 2 weeks, stirring occasionally. Then strain out lavender and bottle in clean glass bottles. May be used as the base for salad dressing.

Lemon-Lavender Pound Cake

3 cups flour
2 teaspoons baking powder
½ teaspoon salt
1 cup butter, softened
2 cups sugar
4 eggs
1 cup milk
½ cup lavender buds, plus tablespoon for glaze
1 teaspoon grated lemon zest
¼ cup powdered sugar for glaze
3 tablespoons lemon juice for glaze

Preheat oven 350 degrees. Butter and flour two large loaf pans. Shake out excess flour. In a medium bowl, sift dry ingredients together. Set aside. In a larger bowl, cream the butter and sugar until fluffy. Add eggs one at a time, beating well. Add flour mixture to the batter. Slowly add milk, beating at low speed until well blended. Fold in lemon zest and lavender buds. Divide batter evenly among prepared pans. Bake 55-60 minutes or until a toothpick inserted into the center comes out clean. Cool the cakes still in the pans on a wire rack for 10-15 minutes, then remove from pans and set on a plate. Make a glaze by mixing powdered sugar and lemon juice. Add one tablespoon of lavender buds. If mixture is too stiff, add more lemon juice. Pour the glaze over the warm cakes letting the glaze drip over the sides. Use lemon slices for decoration.

Lavender Chocolates

2 cups sugar
½ cup milk
½ cup butter
¼ cup cocoa
¼ cup lavender buds

3 cups quick oats

1 teaspoon vanilla

dash of salt

Mix the sugar, milk, butter, cocoa, and lavender buds together in a saucepan. Bring to a boil and boil for 3 minutes. Add oats, vanilla, and salt. Mix well, quickly drop by teaspoonfuls onto waxed paper. When cool, place in sealed containers.

Lavender Bee Balm Bread

1 package dry yeast

¼ cup warm water

2 tablespoons vegetable oil

½ teaspoon honey

4 cups flour

1 cup bee balm flower petals

¾ cup lavender buds

1 cup water, room temperature

1 egg white, slightly beaten

Dissolve yeast in warm water in a mixing bowl. Add vegetable oil and honey and mix well. Add flour and herbs along with the water in stages, beating well. Shape the dough into a ball and place in a clean, greased bowl, turning once to oil all surfaces. Cover with a damp towel and allow to rise in a warm place until doubled (about 1 hour). Punch down the dough and knead on a floured surface for 5 minutes. Divide in half and shape into two round loaves. Place 4 inches apart on a greased cookie sheet and cover with a damp towel. Allow to rise for 30 minutes. Then brush the tops with beaten egg white and sprinkle with lavender buds.

Bake for 45-50 minutes or until lightly browned. A great bread toasted and buttered, or to make french toast with. Use the lavender syrup to pour over the french toast!

Herbal Salad Dressings

⤖ By Caroline Moss ⤕

I often feel I am blessed. I do not have a large or particularly beautiful home, and I do not have a lot of money to spend on repairs and maintenance. However, my little cottage is in the depths of the English countryside, and from my window I have a pleasant view of my small flock of black Hebridean sheep, of my chickens scratching and pecking at the ground, and of the children's pony gratefully tucking into the first of the winter hay.

And most important of all, just a few feet in front of this scene is the little plot that provides the inspiration for my writing, the materials for my workshops, and a ready supply of flavor for my cooking—that is, my herb garden. My herb garden is likely my greatest pleasure—to be able to step out of the back door on a warm, sunny afternoon and choose a bunch of

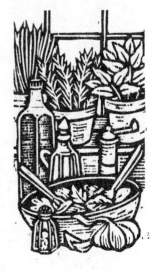

parsley or chives, a sprig or two of lemon balm and a stem of mint; nothing brings me more joy! Most supermarkets still only sell tiny, pre-packaged sprigs of herbs of limited variety. And, when using herbs uncooked in salads or dressings, nothing compares to the use of fresh leaves, just picked from the plant.

In fact, salad herbs are largely easy to grow from seed and therefore very economical. I list below some of the most useful salad herbs and have indicated the life span of each plant. Some are annuals, which need replacing each year, or even several times in a year. Others are perennials, which last, usually, for a number of years. A few, such as parsley, are biennials. These have a life cycle of two years. All the plants mentioned grow outdoors in an English climate. If you have very harsh winters or live in the heat of the southern United States, you will need to check an American reference book for zone suitability. This list is, of course, by no means exhaustive but should provide a good selection to be going on with.

A Salad Herb Garden

Alexanders (Smyrnium olusatrum)

A perennial growing to three or four feet. This is a rather large, rampant plant to be planted close to rougher hedges and walls. It was, traditionally, a vital country food source. The young leaves are excellent in salads and the stems, lightly boiled, are known as "poor man's asparagus."

Basil (Ocimum basilicum)

A warmth loving annual, this plant should be treated like lettuce, with periodic plantings during warm seasons. Indispensable in dressings for tomato salads, the leaves can also be used in mixed green salads. There are many varieties.

Chervil (Anthriscus cerefolium)

A delicate annual growing to nine inches or so. Chevril is common in French dressings and has a delicate, aniseed flavor.

Chives (Allium schoenoprasum)

An easy growing perennial about a foot in height. A lovely salad herb, chopped coarsely with other greens or finely into a dressing to give a mild onion flavour. The flowers are also edible and add a decorative mauve touch to a salad bowl.

Dandelion (Taraxacum officinale)

No need to plant this common weed on purpose; it is everywhere. The young leaves add a lovely, peppery bite to a green salad or with warm, very crisp bacon.

Dill (Anethum graveolens)

A feathery perennial reaching three feet or so. It is usually eaten with fish such as salmon.

Fennel (Foeniculum vulgare)

A decorative, feathery plant growing to five feet or more whose aniseed-flavored leaves give great interest to a green salad. The root, used raw or cooked as a vegetable is a slightly different cultivar of the same family.

Garlic (Allium sativum)

Where would robust, Mediterranean salads be without garlic. Great fun to grow outdoors and use in salads. You may either simply rub a clover round your salad bowl to add a mild kick, or crush a clove and add for a fuller effect.

Lemon balm (Melissa officinalis)

A perennial reaching three feet or so, its lemon flavor is best used uncooked. Too much will taste rather like cologne, but a hint adds a lovely summer freshness.

Mint (Mentha var.)

This is one herb which probably needs no introduction. A rampant perennial to be planted in pots unless you have a large, unfettered area for this herb to grow in. Great in starchy salads such as potato, rice or cous cous.

Nasturtium (Tropaeolum majus)

An annual, growing to 18 inches or so. Its marvellously decorative flower is edible, and its leaves add a hot bite when added to lettuce or other mild salad greens. Look out for decorative flower variations and climbing cultivars.

Parsley (Petroselinum sativum)

Along with mint, this is one of the best known herbs—a biennial that barely reaches a foot in height. Parsley adds depth of flavor, not to mention nutrients, when added chopped to a dressing. Also, add sprigs of flat leaf, or Italian parsley, to a mixed leaf salad.

Arugula (Eruca vesicaria sativa)

An easily grown annual for pots or outdoors. Plant periodically, like basil, to ensure constant supplies, and add to mixed salads for a peppery flavor. A favorite in the wonderful food markets of France and Italy.

Salad Burnet (Sanguisorba rosaceae)

A delicate-looking but robust, foot-high perennial, this little plant is noted in most herb books as having a cucumber flavor, though I personally think you would need a good imagination to detect it. It does, however, make a pleasant addition to a salad that has nothing too overpowering in it; its flavor will be lost if combined with mint or basil.

Sorrel (Rumex acetosa)

A tenacious perennial and wonderful culinary herb, young leaves can be used in a mixed green salad to add a sharp, lemon note. The leaves can be finely chopped and used moderately in a dressing; and you will also find recipes for sorrel sauce, traditionally served with fish. The botanical name refers to common sorrel, but watch for other varieties such as French sorrel (R. scutatus).

Tarragon (Artemisia dracunculus)

A robust perennial reaching two or more feet, tarragon is integral to classic French cooking and gained great popularity in the cooking revolution of the 1980s. The aniseed flavour can over-power but adds complexity if used with caution in a dressing. Be sure to get the correct variety, as named above and sometimes referred to as French tarragon. There is a coarser cultivar known as Russian tarragon (A. dracunculoides) which is not as good.

Dressings

Using the above guidelines and your own tastes, herbs can be added to your own favorite dressing recipes or even to store-bought ready-made mixes. So long as you like the basic flavor of the herb it is really impossible to make a mistake. If you overdo things and feel the flavoring is too strong, simply add more olive oil, mayonnaise, yoghurt or whatever base you are using and keep the left over dressing in the fridge.

Having said that, you should know that one of the best ways to make up herb salad dressings is simply to experiment. I will give you my own favorite recipes in the hope that you enjoy them in your own home cooking, but eventually you will learn that there is a straight forward oil and vinegar base to which variations may be made according to taste and usage.

Herb Vinaigrette Dressing for a Mixed Green Salad

Ingredients

4 parts oil (for a wonderful but heavy dressing use the best extra virgin olive oil you can afford, or use a high quality light vegetable oil)

1 part acid (wine vinegar or lemon juice)

crushed garlic (to your own taste)

a pinch of sugar, or dab of honey

salt and pepper to taste

1 part finely chopped herbs (parsley, chives, chervil, and maybe the slightest hint of mint)

Put all the ingredients into a lidded jar and shake well to mix.

Tomato Salad Dressing

In place of the acid element in the above recipe, use balsamic vinegar. Also, add two parts plain, low-fat yoghurt (this reduces the fat content per tablespoonful and gives the dressing a creamy texture). Don't include any mint but do put in a generous measure of basil if you have any on hand.

Cucumber Salad Dressing

Start with the base vinaigrette, but use only the mildest of acid (white or apple cider, rather than Balsamic, vinegar). Add two parts sour cream, and omit the mint while including dill.

Potato Salad Dressing

Start with the base vinaigrette, and for each cup of dressing add one small, finely grated onion, a teaspoonful of grainy mustard (mild or spicy depending on your taste), and a higher proportion of mint. For a creamy dressing, you may prefer to add two parts yoghurt or mayonnaise.

Cous Cous Salad Dressing

To freshly cooked cous cous, add a dressing of base vinaigrette to which you have added an extra part (giving a total of 2 parts) measure of herbs using equal quantities of parsley, chives, and mint. Also add a finely diced tomato, cucumber, and onion.

Note: Mint is a widely used flavoring in Middle Eastern and North African cuisine. Their favourite drink, other than coffee, is a strong, sweet mint tea made by pouring boiling water onto a handful of mint leaves and leaving it to steep for ten minutes or so before straining and sweetening. Some herb nurseries will stock the strongly pungent Moroccan mint for you to use in these recipes. Otherwise a simple spearmint or peppermint will do as well.

I do hope you try using a wide variety of herbs in your salad dressings, and that you enjoy some lovely herbal meals in your home as I have in mine.

In the end, perhaps you will be inspired to start your own small herb garden if you don't have one already, and you will always be assured of a plentiful supply of fresh herbs at a fraction of the cost of those in the shops. Not to mention the priceless joy you will gain by simply picking herbs or enjoying their fragrance on the light breezes of spring.

A Gala Herbal Breakfast

⫷ By Caroline Moss ⫸

A "gala" herb breakfast can be as grand or intimate as you like. You can set up a romantic anniversary breakfast for two, for instance, or a family celebration for a special occasion. You can follow the theme for a wedding feast, or any formal gathering. The only limit is your own imagination.

The ideas below can be served as an entire menu or picked from as you wish to add a different touch to an everyday offering of toast and cereal. Also pay attention to the various decor ideas I have suggested, as herbs can add simply by their presence at the table or in a decorative vase. You will develop your own ideas once you become more familiar with the versatility of herbs.

Decorative Ideas

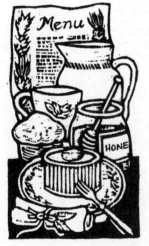

A small sprig of pressed herb could be used on the invitations to start things off in the right spirit.

Decorate with small pots of herbs instead of conventional flowers on the table. These give a country simplicity, though care must be taken when using strongly scented plants such as lavender.

Give guests a herbal memento of the occasion such as a small potted herb plant, herb posies decorated with ribbons or lace, or a pot of herb jelly (recipe below).

Offer herb-decorated menus with pressed leaves or a sprig of something fairly robust that won't wilt too quickly, tied with ribbon, raffia, or twine. Either lavender or rose-mary should hold up well for this. Indicate on the menu what herbs have been used in all the dishes served.

Food and Drink Ideas

These are some basic recipes and ideas to get you started. Next time you want to prepare a really special breakfast, you can do it with herbs.

Melissa Fizz

Serving a delicious, sparkling drink, slightly alcoholic if you wish, in your best glasses, is one way to get any breakfast off to a festive start. A traditional drink in Europe would be a "Buck's Fizz," which is equal quantities of freshly squeezed orange juice and champagne. As champagne is not available everywhere and is also extremely expensive, you might like to try this alternative.

Infuse chopped lemon balm leaves overnight in orange juice, preferably freshly squeezed (use a tablespoonful of leaves per cup of juice). In the morning, strain and mix with equal quantities of any sparking white wine or lemonade. The hint of lemon flavor really lifts the drink.

Herb Teas

It has to be acknowledged that not everyone likes herb tea. For a larger affair it is probably necessary to serve a choice of coffee or ordinary tea in the usual way. It is appropriate, however, to offer one or more herb teas as befits the theme of the affair. That certain herbs have health benefits is now well known, and certain herb teas (such as sage), not having the best flavor in the world, are meant only to be taken for medicinal purposes. The following is a selection of those herbs which make delightful drinks. If you want to plant a corner of your herb garden with culinary (rather than medicinal) teas in mind, then be sure to include: spearmint, lemon balm, bee balm/bergamot/oswego tea, chamomile, lemon verbena, and thyme.

A few points on herb teas in general: 1) They have the added benefit of being caffeine and tannin-free. 2) They can be taken hot or iced. 3) The different herbs listed above can be mixed in whatever combination you wish. 4) Always try to use fresh herbs for tea, even if you use dried in cooking. It makes a huge difference. 5) Sweeten to taste—even if you don't take sugar in coffee or standard tea you may find a little honey in herb tea helps the flavor. 6) As with all culinary herbs, be sure to use leaves that have not been sprayed with artificial or poisonous garden fertilizers.

Minted Strawberries

This refreshing combination of strawberries and mint always add a touch of fun to the simplest repast. You may also, however, want to experiment in combining your favorite fresh fruit varieties with a suggestion of finely chopped herbs. Suitable herbs for fruit include mint, lemon balm, lemon verbena and the sweet, old-fashioned hyssop.

For this recipie, slice six or seven strawberries per person. Sprinkle with a very little sugar to taste, and add a teaspoonful of orange juice and a quarter teaspoonful of very finely chopped mint per portion. Let sit for an hour before serving.

It is nice to serve this in frosted glasses. To do so, lightly beat an egg white in a shallow saucer. Put some white sugar into another saucer. Dip the rim of your serving glasses first into the egg white, drain well, and then into the sugar. Leave to dry.

Eggs en Cocotte

For something a little more substantial and sustaining, eggs en cocotte is a dish of French origin. A cocotte is a small pot, just large enough to take an egg with a bit of room to spare. Should you not have such a receptacle on hand, a small teacup does very well. The joys of this dish are two-fold: 1) unlike most egg dishes it does not need any last minute attention and will look after itself, and 2) each person to be served can very easily be given a choice of flavorings to make their own customized little egg.

For the basic recipe, simply butter your cocottes or cups. Add a large, fresh egg (one dish per person is normally enough as they are quite rich with added flavorings). Add whatever additions, if any, are required (see below). Add a small knob of butter. Top with a couple of teaspoonfuls of heavy cream. Season with salt and freshly ground black pepper. Place all the prepared cups in a roasting tin full of warm water (half way up the sides of the cups) in a hot oven for 10 minutes. Check after five minutes as you want to be sure the yolk stays slightly runny.

For flavorings, to be used alone or in combination, you can choose any of the following: chopped crisp bacon, grated cheese, finely chopped herbs such as chives, parsley, chervil or marjoram, chopped tomato, crumbled, browned spicy sausage, fried onion, chopped bell pepper. These are, of course, merely suggestions, and you may choose to add other ingredients as well.

Oregano and Chive Sausage Patties

These patties add a meat element to the breakfast table, should you want such a thing, and continue to introduce more fresh herbs. To make them, simply take some of your favourite sausages (not too spicy or the herbs will be overwhelmed), remove the skins by cutting each sausage half way through lengthwise and peeling, and combine the resulting pile of sausage meat with a good quantity of finely chopped, fresh herbs. I use about a half-teaspoon of herbs per sausage. Oregano and chive is a nice mixture, but you can experiment according to your taste.

Form the flavoured sausage meat back into sausages or, as I normally do, small patties and fry in a very little hot oil. Broiling will, of course, give a less fatty result.

Herb Bread with Soft Cheese

Rather than serving plain bread and butter with your herbal feast, you can add another layer of flavor. To your favorite bread recipe, simply add some freshly chopped herbs. You can do this too with bread mixes. Both thyme and chives work well, as well as rosemary and marjoram, if used in moderation. Whatever you decide on, simply add a teaspoonful per cup of flour. These herbed breads can also benefit from a tablespoonful of finely grated Parmesan or similar cheese per cup of flour.

To serve with your herb bread, or with plain bread if you prefer, mix a tablespoonful of chopped fresh herbs (such as chives, parsley, chevril, or fennel) to a half-cup of soft cheese. Serve the spread onto small pieces of bread as canapes or pile into a dish alongside your sliced herb bread.

Herb Muffins

There are many recipes for muffins but I favor the following recipe when using fresh herbs.

  2 cups grain (flour, oats, cornmeal, oatmeal)

  1 cup liquid (milk, buttermilk, yoghurt, fruit juice)

  ¼ cup fat (oil, butter, margerine, peanut butter)

  1 egg

  2 teaspoon baking powder (3 if using a whole grain)

  ½ teaspoon salt

  2 tablespoons sweetener (sugar or honey)

  ½ cup optional extras (chopped nuts, grated apple, grated courgette, grated carrot, grated cheese)

  2 tablespoons finely chopped fresh herbs (parsley, chives, marjoram, fennel, thyme, or tarragon)

Beat egg into liquid and fat. Combine all ingredients taking care not to over-mix. Put into muffin paper cups or a well greased pan and bake at 400°F for 20 minutes or until cooked through. A little herbed soft cheese would be delicious served with these muffins while still warm.

Toast with Herb Honey

For an easy way to add interest to honey, simply infuse a plain jar of honey with your own flavorings. Try to seek out local bee-keepers or at least use organic honey. Most honey from supermarkets has been heat-treated to stabilize the product (which destroys valuable trace nutrients).

To make this treat, take a jar of runny honey. Poke in three or four three inch sprigs of an herb. Warm through in a pan of warm water until hot, taking great care not to bring to a boil. Cool the honey, and put the lid back on. Leave for a couple of weeks at which point you can fish out the herb. If giving a jar of flavored honey as a gift, put one perfect fresh sprig into the jar and tie another sprig round the jar with string or raffia. What herbs should you use? I have tried common thyme, lemon thyme and lavender (a particular favorite) with good results.

You will have noticed that most of the above ideas for lovely breakfast dishes were not precise recipes but rather general formulae to be adjusted according to your own preferences and available ingredients. I do hope you have fun experimenting and that one day you serve a memorable Herbal Gala Breakfast to your loved ones.

Get Cooking with Herbs

By Deborah C. Harding

Herbs can enhance the flavor of any meal. A plain salad or pot roast can be invigorated by the addition of fresh or dried herbs. Vegetables and fruits can become taste temptations through the use of herbs. Herbs can be baked into breads, cookies, and cakes to create something special and unusual. Herbs are truly a versatile culinary tool that no kitchen should be without.

Herbs can be purchased or grown and preserved for use several different ways.

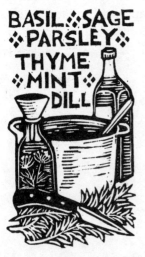

Fresh: Fresh herbs can be purchased at most grocery stores. Herbs are also easy to grow and in a garden or in pots on a patio or on a window sill.

Dried: Dried herbs can be purchased at grocery stores or homegrown herbs can be dried.

Frozen: Pick herbs from the garden or take leftover fresh herbs purchased at the grocery store and freeze. Clean, whole sprigs or leaves can be thrown into a freezer bag and into the freezer for future use. Leaves can also be chopped and placed into ice cube trays filled with water. Use these cubes in soups or stews.

In Oil: Some herbs can be blended with cooking oils, such as olive oil, to be used in cooking. Some of these herbal cooking oils can be purchased in specialty stores

In Vinegar: Herbal vinegars are very popular and can be found in any specialty store. They are very easy to make as well. Fill a jar ¾ full of herb leaves and fill it with vinegar. Place plastic wrap over the opening of the jar before placing the cap on. Vinegar coming in contact with the metal lid will cause an undesired chemical reaction, so care must be take to ensure they do not touch. Place the jar in a sunny window sill for several weeks. Be sure to shake the jar at least once a day. Strain the vinegar through a coffee filter until it comes out clear and place in a bottle or jar with a fresh sprig of the herb. Experiment with different vinegars and herbs. These work well in marinades and salad dressings.

There are also a few very important factors to keep in mind when cooking with herbs:

Use twice the amount of fresh herbs as dry herbs in any recipe. The drying process concentrates herbal oils, making flavor stronger in dried herbs. Most recipes list measurements for dry herbs unless otherwise specified.

When using dry herbs, crush or crumble the leaves while adding them to your recipe. This will release the oils and their flavors.

In most cases, herbs should be added near the end of cooking time. Flavors tend to fade in herbs when heated.

Store dried herbs in a dark area away from heat. Do not store
them above or near the stove. Bright light and heat dissipate the herbal oils, rendering them weak and tasteless.
When home drying herbs try to use dark jars for storage.

The Culinary Possibilities of Herbs

Here are some basic culinary possibilities of a few common herbs.

Basil

Basil is an aromatic herb most associated with Italian and
Mediterranean cooking. It is native to India, Africa, and Asia.
The name basil comes from the Greek word "basileus," meaning
king. In India it is a sacred herb to Vishnu and Krishna. In Italy
it was considered a sign of love. A pot placed on the balcony was
a signal that a woman wished to see her lover. Basil is considered
a protection herb and is said to attract prosperity.

There are many different varieties of basil and most are
useful in cooking. The best variety is common basil (Ocimum
basiicum), but lemon, anise, and cinnamon flavored varieties are
also useful. Basil has a spicy, almost peppery flavor. Leaves can
invigorate veal, lamb, fish, and poultry. This herb works well
with salads, pasta, rice, tomatoes, cheese, and eggs. Try it with
zucchini, squash, eggplant, potatoes, cabbage, carrots, cauliflower, and spinach. Basil is a great addition to soup, stews, and
sauces (especially tomato sauces). Its strong flavor does intensify
during the cooking process. Start out by adding just a bit in
recipes and keep tasting as you cook, adding more accordingly.

To preserve fresh basil, pull off all the leaves from a sprig and
place them on a paper towel, making sure they do not touch each
other. Place another paper towel on top. Microwave on high for
one minute, then reduce power to fifty percent and microwave
at thirty second intervals until the leaves feel dry. Remove from
microwave and let cool for about five minutes. Store in an airtight container. Leaves can be air dried by hanging in bunches in
an airy dry place out of direct sunlight. The leaves will turn black

and it will take about one to two weeks for them to totally dry. Basil leaves can be frozen for use in soups and stews. Basil vinegar makes a lovely marinade for meat and it can be combined with oil useful in flavoring meats, vegetables, and sauces.

Old World Pasta with Basil

Original Italian dishes didn't use a sauce. Instead pasta was tossed with fresh produce. This recipe is one in the old style.

4 large tomatoes, seeds removed, and sliced into strips

4 cloves garlic, sliced

1 green pepper, halved, seeded, and cut in strips

20 fresh basil leaves, shredded

1 tablespoon wine vinegar

3 ounces mozzarella cheese, shredded

Grated parmesan

Pepper to taste

½ cup salad oil

1 pound rotini, cooked per package directions

In a large bowl combine tomatoes, garlic pepper, basil, oil, vinegar, and pepper. Cover and let stand at room temperature. Drain cooked pasta and put back into the pan without rinsing. Sprinkle mozzarella over top and toss until the cheese melts slightly. Add to tomato mixture and toss well. Serve at room temperature topped with Parmesan cheese.

Chives

Chives are a very old herb dating back more than 5000 years. The first recorded account comes from the Orient. The ancient Greeks also enjoyed the mild oniony flavor of chives. Chives were though to drive away illness and it was not unusual to see bunches of the herb hanging over doorways to ward off evil.

Chives can be dried or frozen, but they are better used fresh. Chives add flavor to poultry, fish, and shellfish. They combine well with potatoes, artichokes, asparagus, cauliflower, corn, tomatoes, peas, carrots, and spinach. They also add variety to cream sauces, cheese, and eggs. Add chives to soups and stews or any hot dish right before serving. Their flavor weakens if cooked for long periods of time. Chive butter is lovely on hot bread, and chive vinegar is a great addition to any salad dressing. The flowers of this plant are also edible. Add them to salads.

Chive Broccoli Potatoes

2 pounds potatoes, peeled, sliced, and cooked

6 tablespoons butter or margarine

¼ cup milk

10 ounces fresh broccoli, chopped

1 egg, beaten

½ cup sour cream

½ cup cream cheese

1 tablespoon fresh basil, chopped

4 tablespoon fresh chives, chopped

Salt and pepper to taste

1 cup shredded cheese of choice

Cook and mash potatoes with butter and milk. Place back into the pot. In another pot cover the broccoli with boiling water, let sit for 5 minutes, and drain. Add to potatoes along with the egg, sour cream, cream cheese, basil, chives, salt and pepper. Put half of this potato mixture into a greased 2-quart casserole. Add half the shredded cheese, then the rest of the potato mixture, and top with remaining cheese. Bake at 350°F for 40 minutes. Let sit 10 minutes before serving.

Mint

Mint can be grown by anyone just about anywhere, as it grows like a weed. Mint is a common flavoring in mouthwashes, breath fresheners, and toothpastes because of its clean and fresh taste, and it was treasured long ago by Romans and others. The Pharisees paid tithes with sprigs, and Greeks used mint in their temples and as a remedy for clearing the throat and curing hiccups. Because of its fresh scent sprigs were strewn on the floor in kitchens. Mint water was sprayed about the medieval home to give it a pleasant scent.

Mint was used in the eighteenth century for many remedies, including colic and stomach discomforts. It was also applied to wounds to prevent infections. Tea was used for headaches, heartburn, and insomnia. Placing a mint leaf in a wallet or purse is said to guarantee prosperity. Wearing a sprig of mint at the wrist will keep illness at bay, and kept indoors it will protect the home from any malady.

There are many different varieties of mint. The best varieties for culinary purposes are peppermint, spearmint, applemint, pineapple mint, and any of the citrus mints. Make mint water or mint lemonade by adding a sprig to a glass or pitcher. Peppermint is the best for this because of its strong, cooling taste. Spearmint is a bit milder than peppermint. It can be used with meats, eggplant, beans, lentils, fruit salads, cucumbers, creamy vegetable soups, peas, in jellies, and with chocolate. Flavored mints are a good addition in drinks, fruit, and cottage cheese. Add apple or lemon mint to melon balls with a little sparkling apple cider drizzled over top for a wonderful summer salad.

Mint is better used fresh. When dried, the flavor weakens. Mint can be grown in a flower garden or in a pot. It is better to place in a container as it has a tendency to spread all over the garden. Mint can be frozen or dried. Dry by hanging bunches upside-down until dry and crispy, then store in an airtight container. Dab a bit on the face on a hot day for a fresh pick up.

Vegetable Mint Salad

1 medium red onion, peeled and sliced thin

4 large tomatoes, seeded and diced

1 medium green bell pepper, diced

1 medium red or yellow pepper, diced

1 can garbanzo beans (chick peas), drained and rinsed.

¼ cup fresh parsley, chopped

½ cup fresh mint, chopped

¼ cup olive oil

3 Tablespoons fresh lemon juice

In a bowl combine onion, tomatoes, peppers, parsley, and mint. Drizzle olive oil and lemon juice over top. Toss to coat and serve.

Oregano

Oregano is associated with Italian cooking, and is now very common, but remarkably this herb wasn't popular in the United States until after the Second World War when soldiers came home bragging of the food they enjoyed in Italy. Oregano has a hot peppery flavor. It is used in dishes in Italy, Greece, Mexico, Spain, Cuba, and South American countries. Oregano combines well with eggs in omelets, frittatas, and quiches. It can give new taste to yeast breads, vegetables, mushrooms, beef, pork, poultry, and shellfish. Try it with black beans, zucchini, eggplant, and tomatoes. Oregano is commonly confused with its milder tasting relative, marjoram. These herbs look very similar and they can be interchangeable in cooking, though marjoram is milder. If marjoram is to be used as a substitute for oregano, twice as much must be used.

Oregano's early uses were primarily medicinal. Greeks used leaves to relieve sore muscles. Romans used oregano for scorpion bites. The tea was used for coughs and asthma, while oil was used for toothaches. Oregano is easy to grow and lends itself well to container growing. Snip off the leaves as needed. Oregano can be dried by hanging in bunches. Once dried, run fingers down the stem to remove the tiny leaves and store them in airtight containers. Oregano can also be frozen. Oregano oil can add flavor to meats and be used when making omelets. Oregano vinegar is useful in meat and vegetable marinades.

Lemon Oregano Chicken

4 chicken breast halves with bone, skinned

1 clove garlic, peeled

1/3 cup fresh lemon juice

1/3 cup olive oil

Salt and pepper to taste

3 tablespoons fresh oregano or 1 teaspoon dried oregano

1/4 cup melted butter

In the morning remove the skin from the chicken breasts and rub each with the peeled garlic clove. Place in a china or earthenware bowl. Do not use plastic or metal or the flavor will be altered.

In another non-metal bowl combine the lemon juice, olive oil, salt, pepper, and oregano. Add the garlic clove used to rub the chicken breasts. Pour this over top of the chicken, cover, and refrigerate. Turn the chicken breasts a few times during the day.

Preheat a broiler to high or prepare a grill. Arrange chicken on a broiler pan or on the grill and baste with the melted butter. Broil or grill on both sides, basting, often alternating with the marinade and the butter until done. Serve hot.

Parsley

Parsley is best known for its garnishing abilities, but it is also a very tasty herb. But there is a good reason parsley is used for a garnish. The herb is a natural breath freshener. Just chew a bit of it after the meal is over for fresh breath. Romans placed it on each plate because they thought it would guard against contamination. Early Greeks prized parsley. They would make garlands for use in funeral ceremonies because parsley was associated with death. It seems parsley spouted from the ground where Greek hero Archemorus was killed by serpents. Triumphant athletes where crowned with parsley wreaths since it was though to be one of Hercules favorite herbs. In the Middle Ages parsley became popular as a medication being used to relieve kidney and liver complaints, and to aid digestion. Parsley is a protection herb and is said to stop misfortune if used in purification rites.

There are two differently types of parsley commonly used in cooking. One is curly leaf parsley, used primarily for garnish, and flat leaf parsley, which has more flavor. Both are grown easily in gardens or in containers; both grow well from seed though they are often slow to sprout.(An old saying tells that parsley goes to the Devil seven times before it sprouts; it can take up to six weeks for germination.) Snip fresh sprigs as needed and bring your harvest in to dry before the first frost. The best way to dry parsley is in a gas oven with a pilot light. Tear the parsley leaves from the sprig and place them on an oven sheet. Stir the leaves around occasionally until dry. It should take a few days.

Parsley can be combined with butter and used when cooking eggs or vegetables. Parsley can also be frozen for soups and stews. Parsley has a delightful, mild flavor that blends well with anything except sweets. It is used in Middle East, French, Swiss, Japanese, and Mexican cuisines. Instead of placing parsley on the plate as a garnish, put parsley in your recipes. Parsley combines especially well with all meats, poultry, and fish as well as with any vegetable, rice, or pasta.

Parsley Parmesan Potatoes

1 can peeled whole potatoes or 3 baking potatoes, peeled and sliced thin

½ cup fresh Parmesan cheese

¼ cup flour

3 tablespoons dried parsley, chopped, or 6 tablespoons fresh parsley, chopped

½ teapoon salt

1 teaspoon pepper

4 tablespoons butter

Parsley potatoes are a mainstay of banquet dining. This recipe adds a little cheese for a different flavor. Preheat oven to 350°F. Melt butter in a two quart casserole. In a recloseable two quart freezer bag combine parmesan cheese, flour, salt, pepper, and parsley. Place potatoes or potato slices, a little at a time, in the bag and shake to coat. Place potatoes in the casserole, sprinkle with the remaining coating mixture, and bake twenty minutes. Remove from oven and turn potatoes. Return to oven for 15 or 20 minutes more or until potatoes are tender.

Sage

Sage is very popular around the American Thanksgiving because of its ability to combine with traditional turkey and dressing. Many ancient cultures associated sage with immortality, longevity, and wisdom. It is one of the Native American sacred herbs used to purify and cleanse the spirit. It was also used by the Native Americans as a medication. Sage has many medicinal uses, including fighting epilepsy, insomnia, and seasickness. A legend says that a full garden bed of sage brings bad luck, so it is best for it to share the bed with another plant. To see if a wish will come true, write it on a sage leaf and place it under your pillow, sleeping on it for three nights. If you dream about the wish it will come true. If not, the leaf should be buried in the ground so it can do no harm.

Sage has a pleasant bitter taste somewhat reminiscent of camphor. There are several varieties, but most are not suitable to cooking. Common, or garden, sage (Salvia officianalis) is the best, but pineapple sage adds a bit of zip to some recipes as well. Almost every culture, from the Mediterranean, where sage finds its origin, to Europe, Asia, and North and South America utilizes this herb. The leaves blend well in salads, with eggs, soups, yeast breads, and in marinades. Try adding sage to sausage, poultry, and pork. Of course it is traditional in poultry stuffings, but also try it in pork stuffings. Sage works well with any meat, with tomatoes, asparagus, carrots, squash, corn, potatoes, beans, cabbage, citrus fruits, and cheese.

Sage is a bit difficult to grow since it takes about two years for the plant grown by seed to become harvestable. Sage is a shrub and tends to get old and woody after about three years and must be replaced. Sage leaves can be hung to dry and stored in airtight containers. Dried sage is as good as fresh in any recipe. Frozen leaves can be used as well. Sage vinegar makes a great marinade for chicken or pork and also makes a delicious addition to green beans or beets.

Sage Pot Roast or the Wise Roast

5 pound boneless beef chuck roast

2 tablespoons olive oil

1 clove garlic, crushed

1½ teaspoon dried sage

½ teaspoon salt

¼ teaspoon pepper

1 can beef broth

5 potatoes, peeled and cut in fourths

4 carrots, cut in 2 pieces

2 onions, peeled and quartered

5 teaspoons cornstarch

¼ cups water

Sage is known to be more compatible with chicken or pork, but this recipes highlights its use with beef. In an ovenproof Dutch oven or other deep ovenproof pan, brown the roast in the oil and garlic. Season with sage, salt, and pepper. Add the broth. Cover and bake in a preheated 325°F oven for 2½ hours. Add potatoes, carrot, and onion. Cover and bake 1 hour longer. Remove roast and vegetables to a serving platter and keep warm.

In a cup combine the cornstarch and water. Stir into the pan juices and cook, stirring constantly, until thick and smooth. Serve over the roast.

Thyme

Thyme is probably the most versatile of all herbs. It goes with practically everything, grows easily, and it has a dependable medicinal reputation. Thymus means courage in Greek. Thyme represented elegance to ancient Greece, and was placed in banquet halls before feasts. The knights of the Middle Ages considered thyme a symbol of chivalry. Placing thyme under the pillow is said to ensure a restful sleep. It is also said women who wear a sprig in their hair are irresistible. A legend states that wearing thyme will enable one to see fairies. Thyme was used in the fight against every plague that came along and swept Europe. It was also used as an antiseptic all the way up until World War I.

There are many different varieties of thyme with different flavors and scents (camphor, caraway, nutmeg, lemon) and with different looks for landscaping (silver, creeping, and woolly). The best type to be used in cooking is common thyme (Thymus vulgaris). Thyme lends itself well to container gardening but it is better to purchase a plant rather than plant from seed as the seeds are very picky about their conditions. Snip fresh thyme whenever needed and harvest before a frost. Tie the sprigs in bundles and hang to dry. Remove the tiny leaves from the stems and store in airtight containers. This is another herb where using fresh is just as good as using dried in cooking. Frozen is also acceptable in most dishes. Thyme vinegar makes wonderful marinades and salad dressings. Thyme butter gives a delicate taste to breads, and using it in egg dishes is pure pleasure. Thyme oil is good for browning meats.

Thyme tastes earthy, clean, and faintly clove-like. French cuisine is fond of this herb, and it is prevalent in Creole and Cajun dishes. But practically every cuisine makes use of this herb. Thyme combines well with veal, lamb, beef, poultry, and fish. It is a welcome addition to stuffings and pates. Include it in sausage, stews, and soups. It will bring out the flavor in cucumbers, tomatoes, onions, carrots, eggplant, parsnips, mushrooms, green beans, broccoli, potatoes, corn, peas, cheese, egg, and rice.

Easy Thyme Chicken Pouqui

1 clove garlic, crushed

4 boneless, skinless chicken breast halves

Salt and pepper to taste

Sauce:

2½ tablespoons butter, divided

1 tablespoon olive oil

½ cup onion, chopped

½ tablespoon dried thyme, crumbled

3 tablespoons dry white wine

⅓ cup cream of chicken soup

⅓ cup half & half

In a heavy skillet melt 1½ tablespoon butter over medium heat. Add garlic and sauté until slightly brown. Pat chicken dry with a paper towel and season with salt and pepper to taste. Place in the skillet and cook on both sides until done (about 7 to 10 minutes) Transfer to a serving plate.

In a heavy medium saucepan melt the remaining butter with the oil. Add the onion and thyme and sauté until onions become translucent. Add the wine and cook until the liquid is reduced by half. Add the soup and half & half and stir until heated through. Spoon over cooked chicken and garnish with a little dried thyme.

These are just a few of the wonderful world of culinary herbs used to enhance the flavor of food. They will bring your old recipes back to life with new tastes and vitality in a healthy way. So, what are you waiting for? Get cooking with herbs!

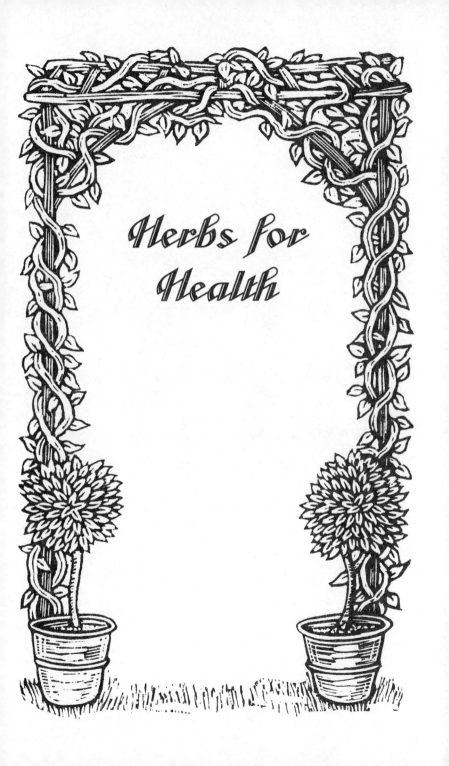

Herbs for
Health

The Best Herbal Supplements

By Leeda Alleyn Pacotti

Every day, we're bombarded with messages about the needs of our bodies. TV commercials exclaim that a certain bread can build our bodies—Twelve ways! And dozens of companies exhort us to take daily vitamin and mineral pills.

Dietary supplements have become part of conditioned thinking in our society. Women approaching menopause and men sensing sexual decline hear about nutrients that will bring their bodies back to a youthful vigor. Entering a new century, we find ourselves inundated by a variety of ideas about our bodies' needs. And expecting health and vitality, we regularly dose ourselves with vitamins, minerals, enzymes, and mega-complexes. As a consequence, we alter our diets, believing pills give us all we need. Behind the modern diet lies an important question: Are these ideas really sound?

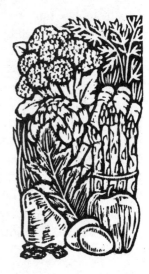

The Evolved Human Body vs. the 20th Century Diet

To answer this question, we should start first at the beginning. 50,000 years ago, humans learned to eat what was on hand. The diet of our ancient ancestors had some prominent features. Meals were simple, with different foods gathered at different times of the day. Foods eaten were recently alive. Edible seeds, plant stalks, even meat and fish, were immediately prepared or cooked. Anything kept longer than mealtime spoiled. Whole foods predominated, insuring humans a full range of essential nutrients when they ate. People ate foods from their immediate environment, receiving necessary nutrients for climatic and seasonal variations. As a last note, food was scarce. People learned to eat by the season or hunt.

About 10,000 years ago, civilization developed agriculture, farming, and herding. Animal flesh and organs were still prepared for immediate consumption. Grain seeds, however, could be stored, provided they were not milled or cracked from their shells or husks. The addition of stored grains, as an out-of-season food, represented a major dietary adjustment, from which the human population is still trying to adapt.

In the last hundred years, meanwhile, food for human consumption has been subjected to high-tech measures. Unlike our ancestors, we follow a very different dietary pattern. Our foods are dead or stale, harvested in different seasons and delayed for consumption through storage or processing. Vital nutrients have been stripped or isolated, specifically to keep foods in a "fresh" condition. Frequently, our consumables are artifacts. Food components, such as vitamins, minerals, oils, and proteins are isolated, and used as supplements. Popular flavors are extracted, synthesized, and processed without the full nutritional spectrum found in the original, whole food. Our foods carry toxicities from chemicals from fertilizers, preservatives, or animal inoculants. We no longer eat foods grown in our environment, but from other regions, even other countries. With technological changes in agriculture, we suffer from overabundance, causing us to overeat or monotonously eat the same foods repeatedly. The modern diet in developed nations is bereft of nutritional foods and their essential components of vitamins and minerals.

The Minerals That Serve Us

Prior to 20 years ago, most of us knew about the need to replenish daily vitamins. Around 1980, commercial nutritionists began to extol the virtues of minerals as basic elements essential for the body's functioning. Distinct from vitamins, most of which cannot be stored over long periods in the body, minerals accumulate primarily in the body's muscle and bone tissue and play a role in organic functions such as enzymatic regulation, utilization of vitamins and other nutrients, and stabilization of the body's systems. Minerals interact with each other in a complicated orchestration of balance. When one or more minerals are depleted, all other mineral balances are eventually affected. Because minerals break down through slow chemical processes, taking massive doses can result in toxicities, causing yet another kind of imbalance. Recently, biochemical science has recognized that the basis of many modern illnesses springs from mineral imbalances.

Within the scheme of nutrition, minerals necessary for human organic functions fall into two groups: Bulk and trace. Bulk minerals include calcium, magnesium, phosphorus, potassium, and sodium, all of which are primarily used in the body's daily digestive and eliminative functions. Trace minerals, of which the body needs very little but which are important to maintain good health, include boron, chlorine, chromium, copper, fluorine, germanium, iodine, iron, manganese, molybdenum, selenium, silicon, sulfur, vanadium, and zinc. The essential requisite for ingesting minerals is absorption by the human body. Most of us have been taught to look at over-the-counter mineral supplements as the most reliable form of ingestible minerals. These prepared supplements come in two forms: Elemental and chelated.

An elemental mineral in a prepared compound is in the same chemical bond it holds in nature. A crude illustration would be a preparation which has elemental or naturally occurring iron ore in powdered form, compressed into tablets or filled in capsules. Elemental iron becomes toxic in the body, because it is not water-soluble and cannot be ionized through digestion. When elemental iron passes through digestive walls into the blood stream, instead of strengthening blood cells, it disrupts their activity. Normal blood cells attack elemental iron as a foreign invader.

Chelation is a process in which the mineral is molecularly broken down. Chelated minerals are then absorbable in the body. However, chelation occurs only when a mineral has an atomic valence in units of two or multiples of two. Some of the minerals capable of chelation are calcium, chromium, iron, molybdenum, selenium, vanadium, and zinc. Potassium and phosphorus are incapable of being chelated. While we might consider pills or capsules to be the easiest ingestion of minerals, plant life abounds with requisite minerals in easily digestible chemical forms. Minerals naturally occur in the soil, which results from accumulations of minute fragments of elements. Microbes in the soil ingest and digest these fragments or salts, breaking down the chemical bond still further. Plants have evolved to absorb these microbially digested minerals. When plants are eaten by animals or directly by humans, the minerals they contain are easily absorbed through digestion and moved into muscle and bone structure for storage and later use. Minerals obtained from plant life allow the human body to assimilate the highest percentage of the mineral. Mineralized supplements must be in a digestible form or else they are attacked throughout the body as invaders or expelled as waste. And ingesting high amounts of one particular mineral causes an imbalance with other minerals or creates toxicity, making the body ill. Clearly, humans have been eating plants for thousands of years and have been able to maintain their nutrition from natural food sources, at only a fraction of the price of expensive supplements.

Eating For Life

Understanding our need for minerals and the foods that provide them starts an exciting rediscovery of how well our world provides for us. As humans, we have long considered that we can "improve" on nature, but in actuality nature is a better provider.

Below is a discussion of each mineral, describing its use in the body, interactions with other minerals, the best food sources, and cautions for avoiding imbalances.

Boron—a trace mineral, keeps bones healthy, builds muscle, and helps prevent osteoporosis in postmenopausal women. It affects brain function, promoting alertness. Boron enhances the metabolism of calcium, phosphorus, and magnesium. Food sources for boron are apples, carrots, grains, grapes, nuts, pears, and leafy vegetables. Boron deficiency is rare. When boron is deficient in the body, any deficiency of Vitamin D is accentuated.

Calcium—essential in bone and teeth formation, and in gum maintenance. It also inhibits the absorption of toxic lead. It helps prevent cardiovascular disease by lowering blood pressure and cholesterol and regulating the heartbeat. Calcium assists the transmission of neural impulses and participates in the structuring of DNA and RNA. In digestion, it activates several enzymes, including lipase, which the body uses to break down fats. Foods rich in calcium include almonds, asparagus, molasses, brewer's yeast, broccoli, brussel sprouts, buttermilk, cabbage, carob, cheese, collards, cow's milk, dandelion greens, dulse, endive, figs, filberts, goat's milk, lettuce, kale, kelp, millet, mustard greens, oats, parsley, salmon, sardines, seafood, sesame seeds, sunflower seeds, walnuts, watercress, whey, yogurt, and green vegetables. Excess calcium prevents the absorption of zinc. When the body receives excess calcium, it deposits the mineral in soft tissue throughout the body, which promotes arthritis.

Chlorine—a trace mineral used by the body as a compound with either sodium or potassium. Chlorine is a cleanser, acting to purify cells, the blood, the liver, and to reduce fat in the body. Chlorine binds with hydrogen, and the resulting hydrochloric acid is a primary digestive juice in the stomach for protein digestion and assimilation of other minerals. Chlorine naturally occurs in cabbage, celery, kale, kelp, parsnips, radishes, spinach, tomatoes.

Chromium—an essential trace mineral providing energy for the body by metabolizing glucose and synthesizing cholesterol, fats, and protein. It co-factors with insulin to move glucose from the blood into cells and maintains blood sugar levels through proper insulin utilization, helpful to both diabetics and hypoglycemics. Chromium is very influential in reducing arterial plaque build-up, found to occur in arteriosclerosis. Foods high in chromium include dried beans, blackstrap molasses, brewer's yeast, cane juice, cheese, chicken, corn, dairy products, dulse, eggs, whole grains, calf liver, dried liver, mushrooms, potatoes, brown rice, raw sugar, and natural mineral water. Unfortunately, refined white sugar and prepared foods, which have high amounts of refined sugar, burn up chromium, causing deficiency.

Copper—a trace mineral that assists in forming bone, hemoglobin, and red blood cells. It works in balance with zinc and vitamin C to produce elastin. It is necessary for healthy nerves and joints and is used in healing, energy production, hair and skin coloring, and taste sensitivity. Excellent food sources of copper are almonds, avocadoes, globe artichokes, barley, beans, beet root, molasses, broccoli, garlic, whole grains, lentils, leeks, liver, mushrooms, nuts, oats, oranges, parsley, peas, pecans, pomegranates, prunes, radishes, raisins, salmon, seafood, soybeans, and green leafy vegetables. In the body, excess copper burns up sulfur, a mineral important in metabolizing fat. When high levels of zinc or vitamin C are present in the body, copper levels are reduced. If copper levels are too high, zinc and vitamin C are reduced.

Fluorine—a trace mineral that works with silicon to harden and preserve bones and teeth. Organic fluorine discourages acid-forming bacteria in the mouth and reduces tooth decay. The best organic sources of fluorine include almonds, beet tops, carrots, cheese, milk, steel-cut oats, sunflower seeds, green vegetables, and natural hard water. Fluoride in drinking water does not have the same molecular arrangement as naturally occurring fluorine and can produce toxicity, which shows as mottling, discoloration, and brittleness of the tooth enamel.

Germanium—a trace mineral that enhances oxygenation to cells, helping the body rid itself of toxins and poisons. It also assists in reducing pain and balancing the immune system. Food sources for germanium include barley, garlic, shiitake mushrooms, onions, and Korean ginseng.

Iodine—an important trace mineral that is essential for metabolizing excess fat. Iodine feeds the thyroid gland to enable its regulation of physical development and body temperature. Without sufficient levels of iodine, the thyroid becomes unhealthy. Iodine also prevents rough, wrinkled skin, and it increases metabolism of calcium. Foods high in iodine include artichokes, asparagus, Swiss chard, citrus fruits, dulse, egg yolk, saltwater fish, garlic, kelp, lima beans, mushrooms, pears, pineapple, seafoods, sea salt, seaweeds, sesame seeds, soybeans, cooked spinach, summer squash, turnip greens, and watercress. Certain foods, eaten raw, can inhibit the absorption of iodine; these include brussel sprouts, cabbage, cauliflower, kale, peaches, pears, spinach, and turnips.

Iron—a trace element that helps produce hemoglobin and oxygenate red blood cells. For iron to be assimilated, the body needs an adequate reserve of copper and chlorophyll, which is obtained from green vegetables. Without enough copper, iron cannot form hemoglobin. Foods containing abundant iron include beets, eggs, fish, whole grains, liver, meat, molasses, poultry, and green vegetables. An excess causes a headache, near the end of the right eyebrow, which is remedied by an intake of zinc. However, a long-term effect of excess iron is the production of free-radicals (incomplete chemical molecules, looking for a bond with another element), which sometimes precursor cancerous conditions.

Magnesium—a bulk mineral that is necessary for a variety of enzymatic activities to produce energy. This mineral assists the assimilation of calcium and potassium and prevents calcium deposits in soft tissue. In the kidneys, magnesium can reduce, dissolve, and prevent specific types of stones. Magnesium is found in most food, but those rich are apples, apricots, avocadoes, bananas, beet tops, blackstrap molasses, brewer's yeast, savoy cabbage, cantaloupe, cherries, corn, dandelion leaves, dulse, figs, garlic, grapefruit, grapes, kelp, lemons, lettuce, lima beans, limes, millet, mustard greens, nuts, peaches, pears, blackeyed peas, plums, pomegranates, brown rice, salmon, sesame seeds, soybeans, spinach, tangerines, tofu, watercress, and green leafy vegetables. To keep calcium in balance, ingestion magnesium at a 1:2 ratio to calcium.

Manganese—a trace mineral necessary for several enzymes to metabolize carbohydrates, fats, and proteins. This mineral is a building block for cartilage and synovial fluid, which lubricates the joints, thus assisting flexibility. Manganese is a brain and nerve tonic. Foods containing this mineral include avocadoes, beans, blueberries, egg yolk, whole grains, green beans, nuts, dried peas, pineapples, seaweed, sunflower seeds, wheat germ, and green leafy vegetables. When manganese is low in the body, sensory perception is depressed or confused, appearing first as hearing and eye problems.

Molybdenum—an essential trace mineral found primarily in the liver and kidneys. This mineral promotes healthy cell functions throughout the body and the development of uric acid, which flushes toxins from the body. Molybdenum is found in beans, brewer's yeast, buckwheat, whole grains, green beans, millet, peas, brown rice, hard water, and green leafy vegetables. Molybdenum also prevents copper poisoning in the body.

Phosphorus—a bulk mineral that is the second most abundant mineral in the body after sodium. Phosphates in the body are involved in each level of digestion, regulated by the prevailing pH level of food eaten. Phosphorus assists in utilizing vitamins and converting food to energy. While calcium is necessary for the formation of bones and teeth, phosphorus maintains these densities by creating the flexible covering over bone and tooth enamel. Most fresh foods contain phosphorus; it is abundant in asparagus, bran, brewer's yeast, corn, dairy products, eggs, fish, dried fruit, garlic, whole grains, green beans, meat, nuts, poultry, salmon, pumpkin seeds, sesame seeds, squash seeds, and sunflower seeds. Phosphorus and calcium need to be taken in a 1:2.5 ratio. When phosphorus is in excess, due to too much junk food, the body can't assimilate calcium.

Potassium—a bulk mineral that has an electrolytic affinity with sodium and activates organs and muscles in the body. This mineral is especially important for the heart. With sodium, potassium controls the fluids inside the cells to keep a pressure balance with the fluids outside the cells. Potassium regulates blood pH, producing an alkaline effect, preventing acidic conditions from the consumption of protein foods. Several hormones, especially those needed during stressful conditions, require potassium for their secretion. Potassium is found in apricots, avocadoes, bananas, blackstrap molasses, rice bran, dairy foods, dates, dulse, figs, fish, fruits, garlic, whole grains, green beans, kelp, meat, nuts, oranges, parsley, potatoes (and peels), poultry, raisins, brown rice, winter squash, soybeans, tomatoes, wheat bran, yams, and vegetables. Continual stress depletes potassium, a deficiency of which may first appear as edema or water bloating.

Selenium—a trace mineral that is an anti-oxidant; it slows or prevents the aging and hardening of tissues. It is a natural protection against mercury toxicity. Men have a greater need for selenium than women, because it is used to manufacture semen. Selenium works well with vitamin E, another anti-oxidant, but it burns up vitamin C. Excessive selenium causes irritability.

Silica—a trace mineral that is found in connective tissue and collagen. Strong teeth, nails, and hair need silica, as does supple skin. Silica has been called "nature's lancet" by naturopathic physicians, because it helps the body throw off accumulations of pus, correcting boils, and hardened glands. It also counteracts accumulations of aluminum in the body, which have been linked to the development of Alzheimer's disease. Plant foods sources are almonds, apples, bamboo, beets, flaxseed, whole grains, grapes, kelp, steel-cut oats, onions, parsnips, peanuts, bell peppers, brown rice, soybeans, strawberries, sunflower seeds, sugar cane, young green plants, and green leafy vegetables.

Sodium—a bulk mineral that is a necessary electrolyte. It maintains the alkaline pH of blood and the balance of fluid outside cells. Sodium, the body's most abundant mineral, participates with potassium in regulating the kidneys and with calcium and magnesium to keep these minerals in solution. Pure sodium is present in all foods and is the predominate and first choice of the body in all digestive processes. The use of diuretics and excessive sweating depletes the body's reserves of sodium. During hot weather, the lack of sodium causes impaired vision, lack of coordination, dehydration, low blood pressure, and, potentially, heat stroke.

Sulfur—a trace mineral that is found in all cells of the body, and in the skin, hair, and nails. It dissolves acids, improving circulation, and generally slows the aging process. Sulfur is found in root foods, brussel sprouts, dried beans, cabbage, cranberries, eggs, fish, garlic, horseradish, kale, meat, onions, radishes, soybeans, turnips, watercress, and wheat germ. When the body is depleted of sulfur, the voice becomes lower in pitch.

Vanadium—a trace mineral that regulates cells in their digestion of nutrients and helps to form bones and teeth. It also inhibits the synthesis of cholesterol. Vanadium is found in dill, fish, green beans, whole grains, olives, meat, radishes, and vegetable oils.

Zinc—a trace mineral that nourishes the prostate gland and normalizes the function of the reproductive organs in both sexes. It promotes wound-healing and affects the immune and endocrine systems. Foods which contain zinc are lean beef, brewer's yeast, cashews, dulse, egg yolks, fish, whole grains, green beans, kelp, lamb, lima beans, calf liver, beef liver, meat, mushrooms, Brazil nuts, oysters, peanuts, pecans, poultry, pumpkin seeds, sardines, seafood, soybeans, sunflower seeds, and tuna. When intakes of zinc exceed the recommended daily amount, this mineral will depress the immune system.

Supplementing For Mineral Depletion

Although nature provides so many food resources for ingestible minerals, our modern lifestyle can easily cause depletions through poor eating and all types of stress. Occasionally, a balanced diet requires supplements. Again, our planet's abundance provides an answer and alternative to over-the-counter manufactured chemical supplements.

Various herbs accumulate high amounts of minerals, making them easily absorbable as capsules, tinctures, teas, or whole plants. When mineral deficiencies appear to be a health problem, the following herbs, listed in order of highest content, help replenish the body. In extreme cases, consult a physician.

Mineral	Herbal Sources
Calcium	Valerian root, Buchu leaf, Pau d'arco bark, White oak bark
Chromium	Hibiscus flower, Spirulina algae, Gymnema, Oatstraw
Copper	Skullcap, Sage leaf, White oak, Horsetail
Iron	Devil's claw root, Chickweed, Mullein leaf, Pennyroyal
Magnesium	Irish moss, Oatstraw, Tumeric seed, Licorice root
Manganese	Red raspberry leaf, Grapevine, Bilberry, Yerba santa
Phosphorus	Blue cohosh root, Bilberry, Yerba santa, Dog grass
Potassium	Parsley, Horseradish, Blessed thistle, Barley grass
Selenium	Hibiscus, Catnip, Yerba santa, Dog grass
Silicon	Horsetail, Eyebright, Echinacea, Golden seal, Ginger root
Sodium	Irish moss, Kelp, Rose hips, Gotu kola
Zinc	Bilberry, Mistletoe, Skullcap, Buchu leaf, Capsicum

Magical Medicine Making

⇒ By Gretchen Lawlor ⇐

Magic is the the art of causing change by powers that reside within us and in the natural world. That these powers are not yet recognized by science does not diminish them. In making medicines by magical methods we are aligning our efforts with the laws of nature in a respectful manner and producing substances with a profound ability to effect change.

There are some basic rules in magical practice which apply to magical medicine-making and use. First off, certain laws of nature must be respected— among them, follow the wisdom of the yearly cycle and the powerful influence of the Moon and planetary bodies upon life on earth. Second, magic acknowledges that whatever one does will be returned three-fold; thus, harmful magic effects a high price just

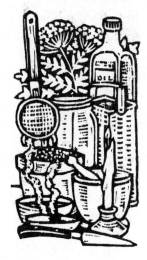

as healthful magic does wonders. Also, magic requires effort, respect and concentration. Its outcome is dependent on the intensity of intention one effects through ritual, meditation, and careful effort. Ritual strengthens, defines, and directs magical power. The wise practitioner will work only for the good. Their tinctures, essences, salves, decoctions and infusions will only be used to restore health and well being. The poisons of the trade will only be used to eliminate that which causes harm to self or another, and never be directed to wishing another living being ill. No medicine will be used which would impair or injure another. Magic is a divine art. You should prepare yourself for the occasion by cleansing yourself and your tools. Keep your thoughts pure and true to your purpose when you are doing your work. A wandering mind dilutes the medicine, while a concentrated, disciplined mind boosts its effect.

Finally, magic takes time. Many magical workings require repetition. There are strong traditions referring to the magical repetition of seven or 21 days, or of repeated dedications of successive New Moons to effect a change. Often the outcome is not instantaneous but occurs in a perfectly normal way.

The Magical Call

The greatest, most potent work in one's life is often that which is unavoidable. Some of us have been fortunate enough to hear an insistent call to some healing technique or method, often out of personal crisis or desperation. From these kind of circumstances many great healers have emerged.

In this way, healers may discover an affinity with particular medicines, which will later go into a "bag of tricks" or a medicine pouch. The work of magical medicine making is the discovery and the cultivation of our magical tools. Consider for instance Edward Bach, the man who developed the first flower essences and from whose work has emerged a whole field of vibrational medicine. His call came out of what could be called a mental breakdown after he left behind a very successful career in medicine and disappeared into the Welsh countryside. The story goes that one day while out walking he tasted the early morning dew from a flower, and noticed an extraordinary shift in his glum mood. From this discovery, Bach developed a series of 38 remedies that transfer the life force of flowers in water infusions. During this life-crisis, Bach's feelings of anxiety, self-doubt, and confusion led him directly to the only healing source in his environment: the particular flower essence he tasted.

In Ireland, where magical tradition has not entirely disappeared, there are hundreds of healing wells, each with the capacity to heal a specific ailment. There are wells for eyes and wells for skin diseases, wells for fertility and wells to restore sanity or hearing or the ability to walk. People come from great distances for cures, a remnant of a great healing tradition in which people in certain regions were known for their ability to heal specific ailments. It was simple, if a person had the gift of healing, often acquired through personal difficulties and experience, then people would take advantage of it. For some healers, their reputation spread far and wide. And there were always the neighborhood healers, gifted with a few plants, or knowledgeable about particular problems. Today, this inclination is once again welling up in society, with the interest in self-sufficiency and need to recognize an inherent wisdom in nature as our medical technology becomes less available to more and more people.

The point of all this is to suggest that each of us has a particular call, often discovered out of desperation. In astrology, this is referred to as the call of Chiron, the wounded healer. Each of us has a personal understanding of the need to discover good medicine to help us heal or soothe any conditions of illness. Magical medicine making is the art of discovering the particular remedies for our medicine pouch.

To Start Acquiring a Magical Pouch

Your magical medicine making starts with the plants you love. That is, you must first use the plants that you know personally. Medicines made out of a personal, intimate affair with a plant are truly magical, possessing an undeniable potency. This is not to suggest the wisdom, the guidance and the ocmpaionship of a good teacher are not important. In fact, the second stage is to begin a study of plants from others through books or lectures, and directly from the plants themselves. But it is best to start with what you already know.

Consider, for instance, the plants that you first knew—those of your childhood. They have been your companions forever, and are worth special thought. They are likely to be healers of early traumas you experienced, and particularly willing to work with you. They are like family. These are plants which you will have no trouble falling in love with, getting close to, listening to. Note next the plants that grow naturally around you, are your neighbors. Don't assume that medicinal herbs are hard to find. Watch the determined plants that manage to live in the cracks of your sidewalk and the ferocious plants that willfully overtake your vegetable garden. These are the plants that want to get close to you, want to be your friends. Get to know them—they may be healing allies.

Herbalists agree that the plants of a region are usually the most potent healers for the conditions prevalent in that place, and that locally grown and made medicines are possibly many times stronger than those procured from a distance. Take care in choosing plants for your garden or your house. Plants can be very protective at the entries of the house, absorb negativity in rooms they inhabit, and act as touchstones for significant relationships in your life. Pay attention to your house plants too, as they provide comfort, oxygen, and negative ions to lift your spirit.

Simple Healing Traditions

Techniques that are most conducive to sensitive medicine making are not necessarily the most scientifically meticulous, even though care and discipline are important elements for the focused intent of medicine making. It is not necessary that a skilled intuitive, magical medicine maker has to adopt the means and methods of the modern scientific medicinal model.

After all, professions have their tools. In magic, we use tools to change matter to magic. Magic is sometimes defined as "change wrought by psychic means," and it is wise to have your medicine making tools chosen and used with intent.

One magical medicine making tradition, the Wise Woman tradition, makes use of an insistent call to certain places, experiences and plants. This school of herbalism returns us to our instincts, to our neighborhoods and to our kitchens—making medicine making a personal, accessible journey of empowerment. As practiced by such herbalists as Susun Weed, who simply espouses working with simples, or one herb alone, we can encounter the subtle healing properties of each individual plant.

In using simples according the the Wise Woman tradition, we become allies with individual herbs, deep friends with the healing properties of each plant spirit. Though there is no exact time frame, once you choose a particular herb you may want to become close it for a year. That is, you will visit with it, sing to it, draw it, taste it, smell it, celebrate its color and shape and strength, note where it is happy and what nourishes it. You will be with it this one herb not just in the day, but in the night, in winter and summer, through hot and cold.

Then, you must keep notes on your friend. You must write about the herb, learn all you can of what others have discovered of this plant. Ask others what they know of this plant. Invite the plant to share what it knows with you. Sleep with it, see what your dreams tell of this plant. If you know the technique of shamanic journeying, use it to travel to the spirit world to gather information about the plant. You must always be respectful. There will be no substitute for the knowledge you gain from this intense experience with this plant.

Another important tool used in magical medicine making is the knife. Some believe your tools should be only those which comfortably hide in your home as ordinary objects. This comes from times when it was not safe to show a familiarity with herbs and healing, in case one would be persecuted as a witch. Other traditions feel that all tools should be purchased and kept only for your plant work. Do what feels comfortable for you, remembering that your preparation and focus of intent is what makes your medicines potent.

In any case, treat your knife with respect. You may wish to dedicate it to your magical work. If so, the Full Moon is the traditionally the time to consecrate/dedicate tools of power. At the very least, wash your knife and ask that it be of service to you in your magical work. If you want to be more ceremonial in the dedication of your knife, you may wish to design a ritual incorporating the four elements. This is traditional magic and can be accomplished with the use of a candle, the flame of which represents fire, a pot of earth for earth, a bowl of water for water, and incense for air. A magical knife is similar to the athame of magical workings, though the athame may be a separate tool used only for energy work. Iron is not acceptable for the blade—stainless steel with a wooden handle is best. Pass the knife through the four elements and ask for their guidance and protection. Dedicate your tool to the highest good.

Other essentials tools include: containers for storage such as canning jars with lids, a mortar and pestle, a grater, a strainer (referred to as a "philtre" in old magical texts), a number of "infusers," olive oil, vodka or brandy, and small storage bottles. All tools for magical medicine making should be purified by washing before initial use, and preferably dedicated and set aside in some ceremonial manner in order to focus intent.

Harvesting Herbs for Magic

A most important step in the work of magical medicine making is to collect only organic or wild plants which display rich color, deep aroma, and healthy growth. After all, the medicine can never be any better that the quality of the herbs you begin with. Harvest only in areas where the plant grows in abundance, and leave without showing noticeable evidence you have been there. Pick from a diversity of plants, never devastate an area, take as little easy necessary for your use. Wild crafting without conscious concern has decimated natural supplies of many previously common herbs. In other parts of the world where there is not as much open space, particularly in Europe and England, the traditions of homeopathy and flower essences are preferred due to the minimal amount of original plant material required for making the medicine. In these traditions, harvesting may consist primarily of a recurring pilgrimage to the plant to visit, observe, share connections and familiarity with the plant spirit.

In all cases be sure to make a positive identification of the plant. Field guides are usually better for identification, herbals are better once you have identified the plant. Some people find photographic guides easier to use, some prefer those with line drawings. Once you have picked the plant, always leave something as exchange. This could be something tangible—a crystal, a stone, tobacco or cornmeal, seaweed or plant food. Or it could be intangible—a prayer or blessing, a meditation or expression of thanks for the sharing of power by the plant and yourself. Ask permission to take the plant's medicine away, and let the plant spirits know what the intent of your workings are. Wise medicine makers plant seeds, particularly in the fall, to ensure the recycling of life energy.

You are always at your best when you are having fun with life. Fall in love with a plant, play with it, dance and sing to it. Loosen your expectations and education, open your senses and allow the plants to become friends. Magic is a joyous celebrating and merging with the life force. Laughter and singing, poetry, music and dance have their place in magical medicine making.

As for when to harvest, there are a multitude of rules. Simply put, harvest the plants you want when the energy you want is most concentrated. Roots are the part of the plant that store energy in the form of sugar, starch, and medicinal alkaloids in the cold or dormant months. Harvest them when the above-ground part of the plant has died back. Leaves process energy to nourish roots and flowers; pick them when they are at their most lush before the flowers have formed and in the morning after the dew has dried and before the midday sun wilts them. Flowers are the sexual organs of the plant, pick them when they are in full bloom, before they form seeds and before the bees visit them. Seeds are more sturdy than flowers and therefore have a longer window of time for harvesting. Pick them while they are still green, before they break up and are invaded by insects. Bark, including inner bark and root bark, can be harvested at any time but are considered most potent in spring and fall.

Once harvested, deal with the plants right away. Allowing the cut plants to lie around dissipates their vital force and encourages mold and hardening. Wash roots to clean off dirt before it hardens. Cut up roots while they are soft. If you are making a tincture or oil, cover them with alcohol or oil as soon as possible. If you are going to dry herbs, separate them and bunch them to dry so the air can circulate without causing mold.

The Timing of Magical Medicine Making

There are many traditions of timing for magic that have been used for hundreds of years. Magic however, needs to be practical. Intent is more powerful than the hour of the day or the day of the week or the phase of the Moon. In all of these systems there is the wisdom of cycles. Notice them and live them when you can, but do not make yourself slave to them.

The Moon is the most important cyclical object to consider, as she influences the tides of life force in all living things. The plant world is intimately connected with the Moon's phases, as the waxing of the Moon brings raises all liquids—from sap in plants to ocean tides. Germinating occurs during this two-week period from the New Moon until the Full. During the waxing Moon the vital energy of the plant flows upwards into the leaves, stalks, and flowers. The waning Moon is a two week period from Full to New Moon when its light is decreasing. This is the time when the vital force of the plant travels down to the roots.

In all magical medicine making, if we want a plan to run smoothly its implementation must be begin immediately after the New Moon. If something is to be removed, or its influenced diminished, the waning Moon is most auspicious. Gather herbs used to remove disease, such as antiseptics, expectorants, and astringents, in the waning Moon.

Another possible influence on the magical workings of herbs are the days of the week. These are each designated in magic to the making of medicines for specific purposes:

Sunday—dedicated to the Sun. Remedies increase vitality, purposefulness, leadership, action, strengthening self image and self confidence.

Monday—dedicated to the Moon. Remedies for issues of fertility, women, for family well-being, and to develop the intuition, imagination, and other psychic faculties.

Tuesday—dedicated to Mars. Remedies increase force, courage, and vitality, and strengthen the sexual organs and libido. Useful when there is inertia or apathy or suppressed emotions that need to be released.

Wednesday—dedicated to Mercury. Remedies increase mental function, clarity, and efficiency. Remedies made on this day are also most appropriate for treatment of the nervous system.

Thursday—dedicated to Jupiter. Remedies lift the mood, add optimism and leadership, and assist in manifestation. Remedies allow one to see new options and horizons.

Friday—dedicated to Venus. Remedies encourage love, harmony, and attraction, and add social grace. This is the best day to make remedies to increase one's artistic gifts and aesthetic sensitivities. Also good for medicines for the skin, kidneys, throat, and urinary system.

Saturday—edicated to Saturn. Medicines on this day are for grounding, for strengthening bones and intention, for assistance in completing projects and for translating ideas into action.

For the dedicated magical medicine maker, there are even specific hours of the day in which to commence one's medicine making. Llewellyn's *Perpetual Planetary Hour Book* lists the local times of the planetary hours day and night for most locations in the United States.

Magic Is Intent

The most important factor in all medicine making is intent. You must focus your vision on the thing that you wish to happen. That is, visualization of outcome is important. Ambivalence or distraction will weaken the outcome of the work.

Fortunately, in magical medicine making, one works not only with one's personal energies but with the power of the plant as well. The addition of one's own energies intensifies the medicine, but to a certain extent one can be carried along by the life force of the plant. Truly great medicine making is the synergetic union of both the plant force and the human intent. The peak of magical work is when one's own powers act as a booster or charger to intensify and accentuate the forces of nature inherent in the plant. If you do not trust, have faith in your work, nothing will happen.

The art of making herbal preparations is fascinating and complex. For those inclined to meticulous technique there are many good resources for herbal medicine making, such as: *The British Herbal Pharmacopoeia*, *The Holistic Herbal* by David Hoffman, any of Michael Moore's herbals, Susun Weed's *Wise Woman* series, and *A Modern Herbal* by Maude Grieve.

For most magical medicine making, simple technique suffices. Magical medicines come in three forms: water based-forms such as teas, infusions, flower essences, decoctions and baths; alcohol-based forms such as homeopathic tinctures and essences; and oil-based forms such as salves, ointments, and essential oils. Most magical medicine making starts with teas and tinctures; flower essences, salves and oils are the next stage.

Water is the best tool for extracting and make accessible a plant's full range of vitamins, minerals, and nutrients. A general guideline is that teas and infusions can be made by pouring one pint of boiling water onto one ounce of finely chopped dried herb in a warmed pot. Cover and let steep for 10-15 minutes, then strain. Stored in a covered container, such infusions should keep for three to four days in a refrigerator.

Flower essences are made by exposing a bowl of freshly picked flowers floating in water to sunlight for several hours, then straining and preserving the mixture in an equal amounts of brandy. This is a system of medicine that comes out of the ancient symbolic language of flowers, and has particular application to the healing of emotional states.

Tincturing is a very effective way of gathering and preserving the active oil-soluble constituents of a plant. There are many complex ways of doing this, though it is sufficient to pack the chopped up fresh herbs in brandy or vodka, store it in the dark for anywhere from a week to three months, then strain it off through cheesecloth.

Oils or salves are easily made by immersing the chopped up fresh herb in a prewarmed fixative such as olive oil or lanolin. The mixture is heated to extract the active constituents. Then, filter the still warm mixture and place in a storage container, allowing it to cool completely.

Perfect Alignment with Nature

The study of magic for anyone desiring to be a healer is not for the purpose of wielding power, but rather to understand and respect the wisdom inherent in nature. Magic is a natural art, born over centuries out of a response to the limitless powers of nature. Magic shows us how to work in alignment with the flow of life to bring about necessary changes. Making our medicines in such a conscious, respectful manner, with a knowledge of correct tools, of perfect timing in alignment with Moon, stars, and seasons, and with a reverence for the plant kingdom makes for potent medicines for the tranformative healing of body, mind and spirit.

Herbs for Pets

By Marguerite Elsbeth

Many moons ago, before humans were created, the earth resembled a giant turtle drifting in an ocean of water. The sky was made of solid rock, and Turtle Island was suspended from the heavens by four cords—each in one of the four directions we know as east, west, north and south.

All was dark, and the animals living on Turtle Island were very tired of not being able to see anything, so one day they caught the Sun and placed it on a great, circular path directly overhead. This way, the Sun would journey across the island every day from east to west, granting them heat and light. Upon seeing this, the Great Spirit told the animals and plants to remain awake for seven nights. However, only a few of them were able to stay awake for that long.

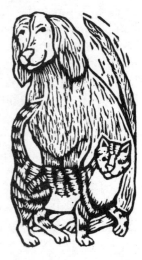

The animals who held the vigil, such as the owl and panther, were rewarded with the power to see in the dark. The plants, meanwhile, who stayed awake, such as cedar, pine, spruce, and laurel, were allowed to remain green all year round and to provide the best medicines for healing. The Great Spirit scolded all the other trees and plants, saying: "You shall lose your hair every winter, because you did not stay awake for seven days."

Finally, humans came to Turtle Island. Although people were last, after the animals, the Sun and the plants, their numbers increased so quickly that they threatened to overrun the land. Therefore it was decided that women would bear only one child a year, and this is the way it has been ever since.

The Way It Was

Creation myths and stories from all over the world tell us that plants and animals were present at the beginning of time, long before the arrival of humans, and that man descended from the plant and animal kingdoms. Such ideas were even held by ancient mystics and scholars in the Western world—such as Pythagorus, the ancient Greek philosopher well known for his geometric interpretation of the universe, who suggested that evolution took place in the following manner, "First the stone, then the plant, then the animal, then the man; after man—the Creator." These beliefs may be the reason why plants and animals are sacred to a variety of cultures even today.

For instance, the people of Wetar Island (between New Guinea and Celebes) believe that they are descended from wild pigs, serpents, crocodiles, turtles, dogs, or eels. Among the Omaha Indians of North America, men having an elk as their totem animal, or red maize (corn) as their plant familiar, can not eat them without going mad. Tribal cultures embracing a totemic tradition believe that to eat of a sacred plant or animal will produce extreme sickness and cause their descendants to die out. Ideas such as these also stem from the fact that plants and animals are our elders, and have much to teach us regarding the ways of the world. Therefore, many tribal peoples have great respect for these creatures, and on harvesting or killing a plant or animal for food or medicine, they always propitiate the spirit of the slain creature with prayers and offerings.

Our interest in both the spiritual and magical roles of plants and animals has grown over the past several years. I believe that this is due, in part, to the ever-increasing list of endangered species, including us. Consider, for example, that the South American rain forest, our main source of oxygen and home to thousands of medicinal plants, exotic birds and animals, and aboriginal tribes, is being destroyed for so-called civilized products, such as the containers used to hold fast food items. The Siberian wilderness is currently being plundered in order to harvest its timber and mineral resources. Nuclear waste is buried in the earth, despite the devastating effect this will have on future generations. Therefore, those of us who are sensitive to both the cause and effect of such atrocities are trying to get back to basics by adopting various earth-based traditions—working with herbal remedies and discovering our animal totems.

Sacred Herbs

Prior to modern medical technology, with its predilection for chemical-based, pharmaceutical drugs, plants were our primary remedial resource. Cultures around the world have long traditions of herbal medicine that are intertwined with astrology, superstition, spiritual beliefs, and customs. Plants have been used for centuries in conjunction with magic to heal, purify, and strengthen the body, mind, and emotions.

Plants respond to our thoughts and feelings just as our immune systems do. This occurs because plants are sentient beings, animated by the same universal, life-giving spirit that ensouls all creatures and things. Known by many names—Life-breath, Great Spirit, God and Goddess—this innate spirit energy is both the healer and the medicine. Plants are sympathetic to our bodies, just as we are sensitive to their healing properties.

And while the scientific approach to herbs, known as pharma-cognosy, determines the chemical constituents and active ingredients in plants, the natural approach to herbal healing remains purely empirical, its foundation based on practical experience rather than rational, established laws and principles.

Contemporary herbalogists tend to eschew the term sympathetic magic in favor of a philosophy called "vitalism." Vitalism is the belief that the life-force inherent in all living organisms is caused and sustained by a vital principle that is distinct from all chemical and physical forces, and that life is, in part, self-determining and self-evolving, as opposed to mechanical in nature. The vital principle of vitalism is that the life-giving spirit—the original life-breath animating all creatures and things—once again makes sympathetic the operative word when it comes to stimulating the healing system with medicinal herbs.

When thinking in terms of the physical body, the word sympathetic is associated with that part of the primal nervous system originating in the small of the back and the chest areas of the spinal cord. The operating faculties of these two areas of the body include the regulation and character of the muscles, the heart, and the glands. It is also associated with a specific nerve of the sympathetic nervous system. This nerve is one of two cords connecting a mass of nerves, called ganglia, along the spinal column, and serves as a base from which impulses for both ordinary and super-sensory perceptions are transmitted to the senses.

Sympathetic emotions are physical reactions caused by vibratory frequencies we can instinctually feel from a person, place, or thing that we are in natural harmony with. Our spontaneous understanding of how the body, mind, and spirit works led to the development of sympathetic magic, and the art and practice of sympathetic magic envelopes two principle ideas: that like attracts like; and that once initial contact has been made things continue to act on one another at a distance.

This first idea indicates that if we can absorb a quality or substance, we can inherit its essential energy. The second tells us that whatever we do to a quality or substance will affect a person, place or thing in proximity to that quality or substance in like manner. Therefore, by choosing to follow an empirical philosophy regarding herbal remedies, we need not concern ourselves about the processes involved or why these medicines work to keep us healthy and fit. The bottom line is, we believe the plant spirits will cure what ails us because we are recipients and witnesses to their curative properties.

Animal Spirits

According to Raining Bird of the Cree tribe, "Each animal has its own Master Spirit which owns all the animals of its kind...all the animals are the children of the Master Spirit that owns them." Animals have an essential spirit energy, just as stones, plants, and people do. When the essential spirit energy in a particular animal is in harmony with our own, we find ourselves drawn to that animal, or the animal is attracted to us. Sympathetic magic and the law of attraction are also the fundamental principles behind awakening to your animal spirit totems.

Ordinarily, domesticated animals such as horses, dogs, and cats, are not considered totem animals because they are tame versions of their counterparts in the wild. However, every animal, including domestics, has its own talent, medicine, magic, and power, and if you've been adopted by a dog or cat you are being presented with an opportunity to learn from that animal.

We identify with certain animals because they speak to and resonate with an intangible something deep in our souls. Relationships we develop with our pets usually entail extraordinarily close bonds based on love, friendship, trust, and respect. Over time, our pets come to know us, and we come to understand the animal's point of view—its likes, dislikes, and behavioral patterns. This association is a mutual agreement, and we should eschew the idea of pet ownership. We are not the masters of our pets; rather, because pets are at our mercy for their survival, we are at their service when it comes to being responsible for fulfilling all their basic needs of companionship, nutrition, fitness, and health care.

Our pets may not be wild, yet health-wise we still need to treat them as such. Nutritional studies indicate that a diet of cooked or canned foods causes the development of chronic degenerative diseases and premature death in domesticated animals. The natural vitality of our pets is seriously undermined by processed foods, chemical additives, and drugs. Coyotes and wolves, the original, true dogs, do not grill or smoke their prey, nor do they journey to the local supermarket to buy dry kibble, canned meat, or artificial treats. Feeding our pets a commercial diet is tantamount to our attempting to subsist on fast food hamburgers and birthday cake.

Feral dogs and cats remain healthy by eating whole animal carcasses. Dogs and cats who hunt and kill in the wild consume the entire animal—hair, whiskers, toenails and all. More than likely, the victim has dirt on its coat, as well as grains and herbs in its stomach, providing roughage and minerals in addition to the protein found in the meat. These fresh, raw foods contain the highest level of enzymes, which assist in digestion. All carnivorous animals require the enzymes, amino acids, herbs and other nutrients found in raw meat in order to remain physically fit, and the closer you come to this ideal for pet dogs and cats, the better. Birds, reptiles, and aquatic critters also thrive from a natural food diet.

My cat companion, Prakriti, is a prime example of the above nutritional perspective. Several years ago, Prakriti developed a severe case of pancreatitis, meaning an inflammation of the pancreas. The pancreas has two functions: it produces digestive enzymes and insulin. Therefore, this ailment is also related to diabetes. Both pancreatitis and diabetes are a result of overeating and long term poor nutrition. Despite all the vitamin and herbal supplements I take to ensure good health, I did nothing to help Pakriti's nutrition. And in fact, she was barely hanging on to life. She vomited up undigested food many times a day; she was dehydrated, listless, depressed, grouchy, and weak. Her beautiful coat had lost its sheen, and I was losing sleep. Desperate to find a solution, I initially brought her to an allopathic veterinarian, who suggested exploratory surgery. This was out of the question, considering her age and condition. Then, I turned to extensive research of her symptoms and stumbled upon the aforementioned ailment. A trip to see a veterinary doctor who also employed acupuncture and natural, herbal remedies confirmed my diagnosis.

This doctor was the first to recommend a raw food diet, with the addition of a variety of herbal supplements. Basically, I learned to prepare what I like to refer to as *Recon-Mouse*. Soon, my kitty was regularly eating a blended pulp of fresh, raw chicken or beef, organic oat bran, sprouts, carrot, zucchini, garlic, and soy sauce. She also received sea kelp, spirulina, burdock root, caraway, comfrey, echinacea, golden seal, nettle, psyllium seeds, rosemary, slippery elm, stevia, and valerian root, bovine colostrum, acidophilus, chlorophyll, and charcoal. She is now twenty years old, and the picture of good health. It required several months of dedication on my part, yet sickness and old age have been replaced with youth, beauty, vim, and vigor. Our veterinarian tells me she may live to be thirty, which is actually the normal lifespan of a healthy cat. I should be so lucky.

Following that learning-experience, my dogs are now fed on organic pet foods, raw bones, and a goodly dose of appropriate herbs, while my solitary goldfish receives an insect or two every now and again to supplement its diet of organic flakes.

If our pets are to return to wellness and stay that way, they require food that strengthens the immune system. This entails a diet resembling what they would get in the wild, along with herbal supplements.

Herbs for Pets

Animals respond extremely well to the healing benefits of herbs because they are, in general, closely in tune with nature; they do not think about the healing process, they just do what comes naturally. Animals instinctively know what they need to remain well, which is why, for example, dogs and cats will eat grass when their stomachs are upset. Our perceptions may conclude that grass-eating causes regurgitation, therefore ingesting grass is bad because it makes the animal sick. However, like fever, regurgitation is nature's way of ridding the body of toxins in the system. Fever and regurgitation are ways in which the immune system rallies to defend itself against unnatural intrusions.

Herbs work to strengthen the immune system by allowing it to heal itself. They do not suppress the symptoms of illness; instead, herbs encourage good health by employing the body's own natural defenses. Should you decide to administer herbs to your pet, keep in mind that while some improvement may be noticed right away, most herbal remedies may take four weeks or longer to get into the system and reveal their beneficial effects.

Large animals such as horses, cows, and dogs require an adult dosage of the herbs listed below. Small pets such as cats, guinea pigs, and rabbits require half the adult dosage. Birds, rodents, fish, and reptiles require two drops of a liquid formula placed in their drinking water. Be sure to replace water daily.

The following herbs are safe for treating these ailments among most domestic animals and common household pets:

Acrimony: Restlessness, excitability

Aspen: Unknown fears

Beech: Intolerant behavior

Burdock root: Stomach and intestinal upsets

Caraway: Digestive problems

Centaury: Over submissiveness

Cerato: Distraction

Cherry plum: Cruelty, abuse

Chestnut, red: Repetitive mistakes, refusal to learn, stubbornness, separation anxiety

Chicory: Insecurity, abandonment issues

Clematis: Sluggishness, sensitivity to noise

Comfrey: Intestinal mucous, internal hemorrhaging

Crab apple: Blood impurities

Echinacea: Fungus and yeast infections

Elm: Lack of stamina and endurance

Five flowers: All emergencies (especially good for birds)

Flax: Brittle bones, dull coat, dandruff, dry skin, sluggish blood, malignant tumors

Garlic: Infectious and inflammatory conditions

Gentian: Lack of confidence, doubt, despair

Golden seal: Infectious and inflammatory conditions

Gorse: Apathy and misery

Heather: Behavioral problems

Holly: Bad temperament

Honeysuckle: Homesickness

Hornbeam: Lack of energy and enthusiasm

Impatiens: Impatience, impulsiveness, and hyperactivity

Larch: Inferiority and hesitation

Mimulus: Fearfulness

Mustard: Depression

Nettle: Poor digestion

Oak: Exhaustion, overwork, over-exertion

Olive Leaf: Stress, mental and physical burnout

Pine: Nervousness, excessive preening, licking, and such

Rock rose: Panic, terror, trembling, fear

Rock water: Joint problems such as arthritis, hip dysplasia

Rosemary: Obesity

Scleranthus: Mood swings, lack of concentration, restlessness, travel sickness

Slippery elm: Excessive vomiting, irritable throat

Star of bethlehem: Birthing, shock

Stevia: Fungal and yeast infections

Sweet chestnut: Fear of the dark, emotional anguish

Valerian: Insomnia, nervousness, panic

Vervain: High strung and strong willed temperaments

Vine: Intimidation tactics such as growling, snarling, snapping

Walnut: Change such as relocation, new environment

Water Violet: Loneliness, shyness

Wheatgrass: Cancer, detoxification, all purpose healer

White Chestnut: Confusion, nervous tension

Wild Oat: Fear, panic, anxiety

Wild Rose: Lack of interest or effort, lifelessness, fatigue

Willow: Anti-social behavior (due to joint pain)

Preventative Medicine

Finally, use these common-sense, preventative measures to keep your pet happy, healthy and fit. Keep your pet's food as organic as possible, as pets are just as susceptible to junk food ailments as we are. Give your pet purified drinking water. Check your pet's teeth regularly. A lack of desire to eat can often indicate gum or tooth disease. Bad breath can indicate the presence of worms. Groom your pet often. If your pet has scales, be sure to keep the habitat or aquarium clean. A regular dose of fresh air and exercise is essential to good health. Any change in habits, moods or behavior may indicate that the animal is unwell. Please keep a close eye on your pet, and seek veterinary advice if a problem seems to get worse. Love your pet to ensure optimum good health and longevity for all concerned.

Herbs for Children

❦ By Liz Johnson ❦

Raising children is as much joy as it is hard work. Obligations abound—to doctors, teachers, sitters, and sleepovers. When children are ill, getting them healthy becomes a major concern of parents, even in the midst of their harried lives. There are common colds and flus, of course, but there are also health complaints that are unique to children, such as colic and teething pains. What is a busy parent to do?

These days, furthermore, many parents are becoming increasingly unwilling to give prescription medication to their children. There is some evidence, in fact, that doctors often over-prescribe medications designed to fight colds, flus, and other non-life-threatening ailments. The alternatives to allopathic, or traditional western medicine, are numerous, but how can a parent find time to learn which path is

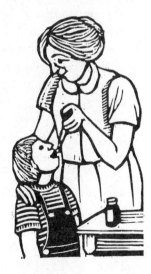

best to take? And, since the descriptions of how these alternatives work are usually written for adults with health problems, not children, there is no way of knowing exactly how to approach alternative healing techniques for children.

Herb Dosages for Children

To begin with it can be difficult to know how much of any herbal preparation to give a child. There are several ways to estimate an appropriate dose for a child. One of the simplest is to take the child's weight and divide it by 150. The number derived from this is the percentage of an adult dose that the child can take. For example, a seventy-five pound child would take fifty percent of an adult dose (75 divided by 150 is .5, or 50 percent). If the adult dose is one cup of an herbal tea, then a seventy-five pound child's dose would be a half cup of that tea.

However, very young children are not merely small adults. Their metabolism runs at a different rate, and this should be taken into account when estimating dosages. Another rule of thumb some herbalists follow is to give an infant (up to twelve months) a dosage one-twentieth of what an adult would take. For children from the age twelve months to thirty-six months, the dosage can be doubled to one-tenth of an adult dose, and for children from thirty-six months to sixty months, or from three to five years of age, the dose would be one-fifth of an adult dosage. In case of any uncertainty, it is always best to consult an herbalist before trying any new herbal remedy.

Once the right herb, or combination of herbs, has been found, the next step is to prepare the remedy. There are several ways to do this. A tea, or infusion, is the simplest herbal preparation. At its most basic, a tea is one teaspoon of an herb combined with one cup of nearly boiling hot water that is allowed to sit (steeped) for five to fifteen minutes before being consumed. Invariably, the herb is placed in some kind of strainer or tea bag so the tea does not have bits of herb floating in it. According to the above formulae, a typical five-year-old would take a little less than a third of a cup of a tea as a remedy. In general, leaves and flowers from herbs generally make good ingredients for teas. Roots are usually made into tinctures or decoctions, but not teas. A decoction is similar to a tea, but the roots are not steeped; instead, they are brought to a boil in wather, then simmered from fifteen to thirty minutes.

If an herbal preparation does not taste good, then a tincture, or a herbal extract preserved in alcohol or other base, may be better tolerated than a tea. The taste may not be better, but there will far less of it to take. Tinctures generally last two years if kept in a dry, dark, and cool place. Herbs stored for tea remain potent for about one year. Young children should be given nonalcoholic tinctures, rather than the standard alcohol-based tinctures. It is also very easy to make a tincture. To do so, simply cover four ounces of chopped or ground dried herb (or eight ounces chopped fresh herb) in cider vinegar. In most cases three cups of vinegar will be used, but the most important thing is for the herb to be entirely covered by the liquid. Place the herb and vinegar in a clean jar with a tight-fitting lid, and put the jar in a warm place, out of direct sunlight, for two weeks. During those two weeks, give the jar a good shake twice a day, making sure that the herbs and vinegar are thoroughly mixed each time it is shaken. When those two weeks are up, strain the liquid through muslin cloth, squeezing out as much of the tincture as possible. Store the tincture in a dark bottle. Be sure to label the bottle comprehensively,—what is in it and the date it was made, and remember that it expires two years after it is made.

A standard adult dose for many tinctures is five milliliters or a hundred drops three times a day diluted in a small amount of water, usually one-quarter cup. Twenty drops is equivalent to one milliliter. A two-year-old would take twenty drops of most tinctures three times a day.

Herbal Remedies for Children

There are many herbs that have been used to help children with their health complaints. The ones covered here are considered safe, and most have been shown to work against the health problems discussed here not only in traditional herbalism, but in modern medical studies as well. Used judiciously and in consultation with an herbalist and a physician, herbs can be an effective tool in maintaining your child's health. For further suggestions, talk to people, especially those who have studied herbs and other parents who use herbs, and continue to read as much as you can about herbs.

Fennel

Fennel, long associated in herbal lore with fire-stealing, has been used to "steal the fire" of colic in babies. If Mom is breastfeeding, then giving fennel for colic becomes easy for the child. The mother simply drinks a cup of fennel tea before nursing her child. Fennel tastes a good deal like black licorice candy, so the tea may or may not be the best tasting tea that Mom has ever had, depending on how she feels about licorice, but the results can be well worth the effort. For those parents who cannot breastfeed, or choose not to, an infant can be given as many as ten drops of fennel tincture in a bottle of water or formula.

Clove Essential Oil

To help children deal with pain of teething, some parents turn to clove essential oil. The fiery essence of cloves is used to fight the fiery pain of teething every toddler goes through. An essential oil comes right out of the plant with no additives or dilution. Essential oils are quite strong and should always be used with caution. Dilute clove oil with a carrier oil, such as olive oil, in a ration of one part clove oil to 100 parts olive oil. To soothe a teething child, simply put a little of the diluted clove essential oil on a finger and rub it directly onto the gums.

Chamomile

There is a second way to help the teething toddler—chamomile. Long associated with the Sun, chamomile bring sunshine into everyone's through its calming properties. If breastfeeding, mothers can drink a cup of chamomile tea before feeding the child. Children using bottles or cups can have a little chamomile tea mixed with water, formula, or juice. And, after a tough day dealing with the hard work of parenting, a cup of chamomile tea can be the perfect thing for the whole family.

Plantain Infused Oil

A popular at-home remedy for diaper rash and other rashes is plantain oil. Made with the cool, soothing leaves of plantain weed (not the tropical fruit), plantain oil can help children with cradle cap, diaper rash, and other skin problems. An herbal oil is made in much the way as a tincture, but it is made with safflower oil rather than cider vinegar. One of the reasons for the popularity of plantain oil is that plantain grows in nearly everyone's yard. To harvest it yourself, consult several good plant identification books to identify the plant. Or you can find plantain at any herb shop. Apply the plantain oil directly to the skin where a rash has broken out. Occasionally a child will be allergic to plantain oil, so watch closely for signs of any reaction. Plantain oil also is said to have anti-bacterial properties. This alone could help the skin heal faster and make it a useful product for daily use.

Burdock

Burdock root is used to fight skin rashes in people older than toddlers. It has a long-standing reputation as a blood cleanser and is taken internally to help the body become healthy enough to repair damage on its own. If a child has eczema, a common ailment of dry, itchy, and sometimes cracked skin, or other rashes, a decoction of burdock root can be taken internally. A standard adult dose of decoction of burdock is one half cup, three times a day. See the dosing information for how much to give a child.

Marshmallow

Children with colds are some of the toughest patients in the world. Fortunately, there are herbs that can help. Marshmallow, with its cooling leaves, soothes the body irritated by coughing and encourages the body to cough in a more productive way, getting rid of the cough faster. Marshmallow leaf can be taken as a tea or as a tincture.

Anise

An herb traditionally used for dry and irritated coughs that tastes a great deal like licorice is anise. Anise has been an ingredient in cough syrups for so long that even in modern non-herbal cough remedies licorice is still a popular flavor. Anise is not only associated with coughs, it also has a historic association with youth. Children often get a dry cough when they become ill, so perhaps the pairing is logical. An adult dose of anise is one to two milliliters of the tincture as often as three times a day. For a child's dose, consult the dosing information above.

Hyssop

Just as there are many kinds of coughs, there are many herbs used for coughs, and each has a slightly different effect on the body. Coughs can range from dry and hacking, like those traditionally treated with anise, to watery and weak sounding. Hyssop is used for watery coughs, like those associated with bronchitis. Hyssop is a mild-tasting herb enjoyed by many that can be taken as a tea or a tincture. For an adult, a cup of tea or five milliliters of the tincture would be a normal dose. Again, see above for the suitable dosage for children.

Agrimony

Another common problem for children when they are ill is diarrhea. Agrimony is frequently recommended for children with diarrhea. It is taken to dry up the stool and to soothe the intestines. Agrimony works for adults too, but is often especially recommended for children because it seems to be very gentle in its action. A tea or a tincture can be used, depending on how the child reacts to the taste. If the child is upset by the discomfort of diarrhea (and who wouldn't be!), chamomile can be added to the tea, or given separately as a tea, to calm the nerves and encourage relaxation.

Peppermint

Peppermint has been considered a cleansing herb since at least Roman times. In addition to seeing peppermint as a cleansing herb, the Romans also associated peppermint with digestion and calm stomachs. It has a reputation for calming the smooth muscle of the digestive tract which contract when one is about to vomit. Peppermint has been used to calm upset tummies and has the benefit of tasting good to most children. Peppermint is considered a cooling herb, and taken either as a tea or as a tincture, peppermint is often used to treat stomach upset accompanied by fever. If anyone in the family is prone to carsickness, having a bottle of peppermint tincture on long car trips can be a lifesaver.

Ginger

Another popular tummy cure, especially for motion sickness, is crystallized ginger. Crystallized ginger is ginger that has been preserved with sugar. Unlike peppermint, ginger is considered a warming herb and is associated with Mars. It is not used as often with children who have fevers, but it is especially popular for children with motion sickness. For children who like ginger, a piece of crystallized ginger can be a real treat! People with gallstones should consult a physician before using ginger.

Healing and Help: The Plants of Hawaii

≈ By Bernyce Barlow ≈

*T*he abundant plant life of the Hawaiian Islands has been used to bring health to people throughout the islands' history. Many of the plants are called "canoe plants" because they were brought to Hawaii on the canoes that carried the people who migrated from Asia, Polynesia, and the outer Pacific Rim. The canoe plants adapted well to the islands and became an important part of the sacred lifestyle of the Hawaiians.

There is a mystical side to the canoe plants. Certain gods and goddesses favored certain plants and lent their assistance through the help and healing of the plant. The *kahunas*, or local shamans, who specialized in healing with herbal and plant medicine were called *la'au lapa'au*. Schools were set up just to study and propagate plant life. Medicine gardens and their secrets

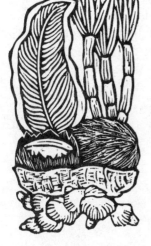

were well guarded. Other kahunas whose specialty was botany made an art of developing canoe plant hybrids.

Ginger

One example is ginger. At one time there were over 350 different types of ginger, or *awapuhi* as it is known in Hawaiian, growing on the Hawaiian Islands, each with its own special use. Some classifications of ginger were used for medicine, other types were grown for dye, spices, ceremony, or to make leis of distinctive scent or color. This hybrid process played an important role in the development of all the canoe plants of the past, as well as those surviving today.

More specific uses of ginger, both past and present, include pounding the dry root into powder and sprinkling it in between the pleat of linens while they are in the closet, much like a sachet. The Hawaiians of old added it to their folded *kapa* cloth to give it a fresh scent. The leaves of the awapuhi are likewise aromatic and are used to wrap food when cooking in the underground ovens, or *imu*. The leaf stalks are also placed in the imu to give certain Hawaiian dishes, such as pork and fish, a distinctive taste and essence. Ginger was used in medicine, too. The cooked, pulverized root was pressed on a toothache to relieve pain, or mixed with sea salt and *noni* fruit and made into a poultice for sprains. The root pulp was also strained and mixed with water or sugar can, or *ko*, juice and made into a tea for circulation and indigestion. Historically, another common use for ginger for cleaning hair and body, as the slime of the flower heads makes a sudsy juice that cleans, softens, and holds a heavenly scent.

If you live in a warm climate or have a greenhouse you can cultivate ginger. It needs plenty of space as the roots are shallow and spread out close to the surface. In the autumn, if you plant a piece of root stock with buds on it in a trench it will go dormant for the winter, then come to life in the spring. Root stock is probably how ginger traveled to the islands. Typical of the canoe plants, ginger likes lots of water and sun. Ask your nursery person what kinds of ginger are available. For example, Zingiber zerumbet is the official name of shampoo ginger. The edible ginger is referred to as awapuhi pake, or Chinese or Jamaican ginger. Although ginger is a fine example of a canoe plant, there are many others for us to explore. Some are listed below for your enlightenment and entertainment. This is not a complete list but a good representation of the variety of canoe plants and how the Hawaiians used them "in a good medicine way."

'Ape: Elephant Ear Plant

Originating from Southeast Asia, the 'ape has huge leaves that resemble the ear of an elephant, hence its name. 'Ape traveled throughout the Pacific and was carried as roots to the Hawaiian islands via Polynesia. It is a relative of the taro plant, whose corm and underground stem can be eaten after sufficient cooking. As with taro, small crystals of calcium oxalate are found in the 'ape-plant, and can only be broken down with thorough cooking. Otherwise, these crystals can irritate the mouth and internal tissues. In general, 'ape doesn't taste very good, and was turned to for food only in times of famine. As a medicine, however, the juice from the stem of the 'ape was applied to skin irritations caused from plants that sting and make you itch like ko or nettles. Kahunas used to make wraps of 'ape and *ti* leaves to break fevers. 'Ape has a bitter sap that is credited for magically frightening away dark spirits.

Growing 'ape is not difficult given the right climate. Moist, well-composted soil is essential, as is a certain amount of shade. The 'ape plant stands three to eight feet high, well below the canopy of taller, denser trees of the Hawaiian forests, so it has adapted to a shady patio environment. Propagate 'ape by planting root cuttings.

Kalo: Taro Plant

The *kalo* plant was the staff of life of Hawaii. It was considered a sacred plant and was a primary food and medicine source for the islanders. There were once over 300 types of taro growing on the islands, each with specific characteristics. Fewer than 100 types remain today. In old Hawaii, *poi* was the main food staple. It was made from pounded taro roots moistened with water. Hawaiians consumed it at the rate of three to five pounds a day. Poi paste is full of vitamins and minerals, and when accompanied with a traditional side dish of fish, seaweed, yams, or fruit provided a good foundation for the traditional Hawaiian diet.

Taro tubers were also often steamed, boiled, or baked with added seasonings, served much like a potato. The young leaves of the taro were cooked as greens, and the mashed roots were prepared as a nutritious food for both babies and the elderly. Pudding-like desserts were also made from the roots. Furthermore, the taro corm was also cooked and consumed as food. Like the ʻ*ape* plant, all parts of the taro need to be well cooked due to calcium oxalate crystals.

The practical and medical uses of the taro plant and poi are as varied as its food value. Dye was made for kapa (also called tapa) cloth from the taro plant. Some kinds yielded a red dye from the leaf stem. Sludge from taro patches was also used as a black dye.

As a carbohydrate, poi can aid against diarrhea when mixed with *pia*, or arrowroot, starch. It can also draw infection from boils when combined with noni and made into a poultice. Taro root paste and sea salt have been known to stop infections, and juice from the leaf stem is said to keep insect bites from itching.

In Hawaii, swapping taro varieties is a backyard pastime. If you plan on cultivating your own taro patch you will need to get hold of a taro corm, then cut a half-inch slice off the top, making sure that it is connected to six to ten inches of the leaf stem, and plant it. Keep the leaves above the surface. Within a year your taro should be ready to harvest. There are dryland and wetland varieties of different tastes and colors. The wetland varieties require a lot of water! More information about tarot varieties is available on the Internet.

Kamani: True Kamani Tree

The true *kamani* tree is a member of the mangosteen family and can grow to fifty feet in height. The kamani haole, or false kamani, is a different plant, and not as useful. It was brought to the islands late in their history as an ornamental shade tree. The true kamani has a long history on the islands, and was probably propagated by seeds brought from the Pacific Rim islands. It is best known for its wood, flowers, and the oil that came from kernels found inside the fruit of the tree. Because kamani wood has no unpleasant odor or taste containers for food and water were made from it. The flowers were exceptionally fragrant and used to make leis and ground into powder to scent tapa cloth. Kamani flowers smell like orange blossoms and their essence was a popular scent of ancient Hawaii. The volatile kamani kernels, also called *punnai* nuts, were strung to make torches and the oil from the kernels, also called *dily oil*, make a terrific massage lotion when mixed with coconut oil. True kamani can be planted from a seed and cultivated in a tropical environment.

Ki

The *ki* plant is a member of the lily family. Hawaiian chants tell us the ki is sacred to the god Lono and the goddess of the hula, *Laka*. It is also sacred to the kahunas and is often used in ceremony. The islanders consider the ki a symbol of luck, strength, and survival, and honor its versatility as a ceremonial medicine plant. A tea made from boiled ki leaves was given to calm nerves and relieve aching muscles. Kahunas placed damp leaves over a patient to break a fever or cure a headache. Steam from the boiled shoots helped to relieve congestion, and the flower essence was used when treating asthma. But perhaps the most popular use of this plant had to do with the brandy-like liquor that was distilled from its mashed, fermented roots. This joy juice was called *okolehau*, or *oke* for short, and contributed to the merriment of many Hawaiian celebrations!

The ki plant also provided many necessities to the islanders. The leaves were woven into a myriad of articles like capes, hula skirts, and sandals. Cups and plates were made from ki, as was the roof thatching that covered many of the island homes. Ki leaves acted as a protective ground covering during ceremonies and as tablecloths during picnics.

Ki plants like wet gardens with loose soil and good Sun exposure, with daily periods of shade. Ki can be propagated from cuttings. If you plant the cutting vertically it will yield one plant. Horizontal planting will yield more than one plant.

Ko: Sugar Cane

This amiable plant is a perennial grass whose stalk can grow as tall as twenty feet high. Ko is best known for the sweet, sugary sap that is found inside its stem. This sap was used to make medicine taste better and to flavor food and drinks. Sometimes the sap crystals were toasted and made into a children's tonic. There are many varieties of ko. The most popular medicine ko is white ko. Red ko is also said to have medicinal uses.

Ko is easy to grow. Dig a six to eight inch deep trench, place an eight-inch section of ko from the upper part of the plant into the trench sideways, bless, and cover with soil. Each node will create a new cane stock. Give your ko plant plenty of water and lots of sunshine and it will sweetly reward your efforts.

Uala: Sweet Potato

Kamapuaía is said to be the god of the sweet potato, a gift to the islanders from tropical South America. Ancient Hawaii hosted more than 200 varieties of *uala*, but in modern times there are less than a handful of these varieties left. In addition to taro poi, uala was another medicine and food staple regularly used by the island people. As a medicine, uala was used to induce vomiting when mixed with ti stem slime. Kahunas who dealt with childbirth made the plant into a tonic for use during pregnancy to aid lactation. Mucus was reduced through a sore throat gargle made from the uala, and if swallowed, it would work as a laxative!

A type of uala called *po* was also used as a fish bait. The weathered vines went to feed the pigs or to pad and stuff kapa mattresses. But it was the sweet potato and its tubers that held the fancy of the Hawaiian cooks, who made this food into delectable delectable dishes similar to many of the sweet potato recipies we enjoy today.

When propagating, use vine cuttings broken off from the last twenty inches of the plant, and keep the cuttings in water until planting. Remove most of the leafs from the cutting but for the top five. Plant in well drained soil. Little roots will begin to appear if you keep the vine well watered. Like most vine plants, Uala takes up a lot of space so plan accordingly.

Wauke: The Paper Mulberry Tree

Worldwide, throughout history each culture found its own unique way to grow and make cloth for covering, clothing and linens, the Hawaiians were no exception. The bark from the wauke tree provided them with material to make a cloth-like material called kapa. To make kapa, islanders would strip the inner bark from certain plants in the mulberry family, and soak it in running water from a spring, stream, or shallow tide pool to remove starches and saps from the bark. When this process was complete, some of the strips were set aside to make fish nets, ropes, and string. The remaining strips were put together and dried, creating a bundle of strips that were stuck together. When a big enough bundle was accumulated, the kapa maker soaked the bundle for half a day, then beat it to loosen the fibers. To make the fibers even softer they were placed under banana leaves and left to ferment for about a week. At that point, the tapa maker gathered the fibers together and kneaded them into a doughy substance resembling a loaf of bread. Finally, the prepared bark was placed on a long, flat piece of wood and pounded with a wooden mallet until a solid piece of cloth was formed. The cloth was then dried in the Sun.

The mallets had symbols and designs carved into them that acted like the kapa maker's signature. The beating process imprinted this signature, or watermark, into the cloth. Each tapa makers distinct watermark was visible when the cloth was held up to the Sun. The Sun-bleached white cloth was like an unpainted canvas to a kapa maker. Hawaiians became well-known for their style and method of tapa printing and design. The colors were deep rich earth colors extracted from plant and mineral dyes. Brown dyes came from the kuiki root bark and red from its tree bark. Red also was harvested from noni root bark by mixing coral into it. Bright yellow came from noni roots and pale yellow from 'olena, or turmeric, tubers. By boiling the young ëolena shoots, orange and gold dyes were made; mature ëolena stems yielded righter oranges and golds. After dyeing, wooden block stamps with different symbols and designs carved into them were used to stamp designs onto the kapa. This style of imprinting, which was unique to the Hawaiian islands, has only recently been rediscoved by modern artisans.

As a medicine plant, the sap from the wauke was used as a laxative and also to cure mouth thrush. Kahunas say if you mix the wauke sap with the burnt ashes of kapa the cure will be more potent. This tree is hard to "beat" when it comes to practical use. Unfortunately there are few left on the islands. The good news is it can be propigated from seed, but the wauke needs a moist, fertile place to grow in the sun.

Canoe Plant Recipies

Glazed Carrots

5 carrots

1 tablespoon Hawaiian sugar

¼ cup orange juice

¼ teaspoon ginger

1 teaspoon Hawaiian salt

1 teaspoon cornstarch

Slice carrots into one-inch pieces and cook in boiling water until tender for twenty minutes. In another pan mix the remaining ingredients and bring to a simmer. Put the carrots into the glaze mixture. Cook gently until the glaze is thickened. Serve.

Uala

one serving of uala (sweet potato)

banana or taro Leaves

1 tablespoon Hawaiian sugar

¼ teaspoon ginger

a handful of dry toppings like raisins and macadamia nuts

1 tablespoon butter

1 tablespoon oil to grease the leaves

Gently scrub the skin of the sweet potato without removing, and putting a small slit in the top of the potato, wrap it in oiled wet banana or taro leaves and tie with cordage. (Tin foil will work as a substitute.) Bake at 350°F until the potato is soft inside—the actual time depends on the size of the potatoes. In a small bowl, mix the remaining dry ingredients. Unwrap the uala, cut and add butter. Sprinkle with sweet potato topping. Enjoy

Fresh Coconut Milk

2 cups boiling water

4 cups grated coconut

Pour two cups boiling water over 4 cups grated coconut, let stand for 20 minutes. Strain, chill and serve

Haupia: Hawaiian Pudding

7½ tablespoons cornstarch

4 tablespoons Hawaiian sugar

⅛ teaspoon salt

2 cups coconut milk

In a saucepan combine a half-cup coconut milk with the dry ingredients until they make a paste, then add the rest of the milk. Cook on low heat and stir rapidly to keep the mixture from curdling. When the mixture is clear, thick, and coats the spoon, pour it into a shallow pan and set aside to firm and cool.

Aloha!

Homeopathy and Magic

By Gretchen Lawlor

Strange Remedies in the Herbal Realm

Homeopathic medicine has been around for at least two hundred years, and is presently experiencing a surge of popularity. This may be because people, discouraged by the inconsistent results and debilitating side effects of many conventional medicines, are hungry for other options.

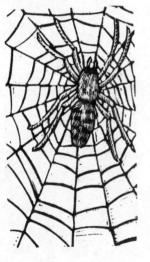

Homeopathic medicines have been tried by over 60 % of American households in the past 8 years, and more and more people are becoming converts to this system of healing. Readily available in drug and health food stores - homeopathic first aid medicines such as Arnica and Apis are becoming common home health tools.

Or it may be in fact part of a bigger trend. In all fields of life these day, as the trappings of society move beyond our easy comprehension, people have begun to consider new perspectives that verge from the mechanistic scientific theories of Newton to the more integrative world view of Einstein. That is to say, we must look beyond the physical body to see human beings as a series of complex energy fields, and we must find ways of healing the complete complex of physical, mental, and emotional bodies in the human animal.

What this brings us to is to return with fresh eyes to an old paradigm—where science and magic are interconnected. For instance, progressive psychotherapists are increasingly making use of astrology in their practice, and doctors are reconsidering the role of sympathetic magic in healing. Homeopathy, therefore, is a rich ground for healing through a perusal of herbs. Consider arnica, which is current popularity in sports injuries and surgical recovery, or apis, made by shaking up honey bees in a jar and mixing them in a blender with alcohol, which is very successful in the home treatment of sore throats. Oscillococcinum, made from duck gizzards, strange as that sounds, is actually a successful homeopathic alternative to flu shots in an era of wide spread, debilitating flu epidemics.

The following descriptions are intended to list a few of the more unusual and surprising—but effective—remedies in the homeopathic pharmacy.

Remedies Made from Poisons and Venoms

Tarentula

There are a number of remedies made from different spiders, but tarentula hispanica, made from live Spanish tarantulas macerated in alcohol, is the most common. This remedy was discovered by a Spanish homeopath named Nunez who mentions an association between this remedy and a famous Spanish dance called the tarentella. Tarentism is a dancing mania, supposedly occurring in persons bitten by the tarantula. The cure is music and dancing, which give a keynote to this remedy.

Tarentula is suited to nervous, hysterical patients subject to extreme restlessness. The restlessness accelerates into fidgeting, quivering, jerking, trembling, and twitching. Symptoms appear suddenly with violent force and uncontrolled movement of the limbs. Tarentula has been used successfully to treat hysterical epilepsy, Meniere's Disease, Parkinson's, and spinal irritations.

Naja

The poison from the deadly cobra has been used from ancient times by Indian homeopathic practitioners, and is gaining popularity in the West. Available and listed in homeopathic pharmacopoeia as the medicine of the naja repudian—the hooded snake of Hindustan—it is made from from fresh venom acquired from snake charmers.

Used in low potencies, it is used for heart disorders, especially for damaged heart tissue, and it relieves the symptoms of infectious diseases and angina. It also helps headaches with severe pains in the left temple, especially those associated with menopause or unresolved grief. In the plague epidemic of 1899-1900, naja proved more efficacious than the more common medicines of the day.

Lachesis

Lachesis is a very common homeopathic remedy, made from venom from the bushmaster snake, or surukuku, of South America. Its discovery was made by Hering, an early homeopathic explorer who suffered excruciating, life threatening symptoms from the handling and preparation of the remedy. Because of his ignorance of the dangers of lachesis overdose, Hering was thrown into a fever with tossing delirium and mania which only subsided over time.

Lachesis is actually an excellent remedy for alcoholic delirium tremens, high blood pressure, manic-depressive mania, and certain kinds of hemorrhaging. It has particular use in menopausal conditions and depression having to do with menstrual flooding.

Wired but Wonderful Remedies

Aurum

Aurum is gold, homeopathically diluted and prepared. For many years, it had been overlooked until rediscovered by homeopathy. Gold has had application in modern times in allopathic medicine as a treatment for rheumatism, though it has even more profound application as an antidepressant. Aurum treats melancholy conditions in the patient, and can even treat suicidal tendencies.

Chocolate

Mayan Indians believed the cocoa tree was a gift from the gods, and that a drink made from the seeds would nourish them after death. In Aztec medicine, cocoa was highly valued. Made from the cocoa beans (Theobroma cocoa) of tropical Central and South America, chocolate helps relieve skin afflictions, particularly itchy skin with dry, rough patches. It soothes a mind rushing from one thing to another, irritability, and aversion to writing, as well as anxiety before meeting people. Chocolate is helpful for clearing discharges from the nose and relieving itching at the end of the nostril.

Spider's Web

Tela araneum, or spider's web, has ancient medical roots. Bandages were made by herbalists from spider webs, which contain penicillin like constituents. The homeopathic form is made from the cobweb of "black spiders found in dark places" and possesses a remarkable ability to induce calm and lower the pulse rate. It brings on a tranquility resembling the action of opium and is helpful in sleep disorders and has no narcotic effect or residual grogginess. In spasmodic disorders such as asthma, periodic headaches, and muscular irritability, spider's web can help bring on a soothing sleep.

Lac Caninum

Lac caninum or Dog's Milk is the most popular of all remedies made from milk. Lac caninum was used by the Greeks to treat ulceration of the cervix, photophobia, and otitis. Homeopathy has confirmed the accuracy of these old observers through the rigors of modern homeopathic testing. Lac caninum works when there are symptoms that alternate sides. It is particularly effective in serious sore throats, diphtheria, and rheumatism. There has recently been considerable homeopathic research into the uses of lac caninum to treat attention deficit disorder. Studies show that when reading or speaking difficulties exist, lac caninum may be an effective treatment.

North Pole

Magnetis polus articus is the homeopathic name for north pole, the remedy made by exposing water or a neutral homeopathic base substance to the north pole of a very strong magnet. Elizabeth Wright Hubbard, an early American homeopath quotes this remedy as causing a complete and immediate cure in a case of painful herpes zoster. Symptoms improved by this remedy are those occurring in the teeth and jaws, including toothache and jaw pains.

South pole, or magnetis polus australias, meanwhile, is made by exposing alcohol to the south pole of a magnet. This cure is effective in cases of ingrown toenail.

Bedbug

Cimex is a traditional remedy made by pulverized bedbugs, and is used to treat intermittent fever.

Pus

Tuberculinum, made from tubercular abscess material, is only one of many remedies made from pus or diseased tissue from seriously ill people. These are very popular and profoundly effective remedies, though the wise homeopath will seldom elaborate on the source material of the remedy to the patient. Recall, however, that the remedy itself is from a highly diluted and processed form of the original pus, with only the energetic imprint of its source remaining.

Tuberculinum is a great remedy for all chest complaints, from colds and bronchitis to the early stages of tuberculosis. Often, furthermore, homeopathic treatment with tuberculinum will stop a restless urge to relocate or travel. Be forewarned if you love to take journeys.

Three more common pus remedies are: syphilinum, made from syphilitic pus from active sores, psorinum, made from the pus from scabies vesicles, and medorrhinum, made from gonorrheal pus. These all have profound effect in chronic conditions which are unresponsive to other treatments. Syphilinum has been used in treatment of cancer, severe types of nero-arthritis, mental disturbances of various sorts, and a number of kinds of paralysis. Psorinum resolves difficult skin problems where all else has failed, and is known for its beneficial effect upon chronic hay fever. It is also effective in treating a hereditary tendency towards alcoholism. Medorrhinum is a treatment for chronic rheumatism, sinusitis, pelvic inflammations in women, and infertility and impotence.

Cannabis

Cannabis indica and Cannabis sativa are both major remedies in the homeopathic pharmacy, though they are unavailable over the counter in the U.S. Interestingly enough, once a homeopathic medicine is diluted and prepared, western science is unable to identify any of the active constituents of the original substance. Cannabis in homeopathic form should therefore be legal.

Tinctured from the flowering tops of the plant, cannabis has been used in treating problems of the sexual and urinary organs—including cystitis—and for treating confusion of thought and speech. It has uses also in treating cases of excessive indulgence of recreational marijuana, helping to clear residue from the system and decrease dependency.

Peyote

Anhalonium, or peyote, is prepared for homeopathic use by cutting up the small cactus buttons from the peyote plant of the Southwestern U.S. into small fragments and pouring on boiling water twice. Medically its chief use is as a cardiac tonic and respiratory stimulant. The mental conditions it soothes have similarities to the states it causes when used in a gross form or ceremonially by Native Americans. This is a foundational premise of homeopathic medicine: that a homeopathic dosage of a substance is curative to the conditions it causes when used in its original form.

With anhalonium therefore, it treats conditions of delirium and hallucination, and it is useful with patients whose mental states have rendered them out of contact with the outside world and with a diminished concept of time.

Cocaine

Coca was considered a divine plant by the Incas. It was used as an intoxicant for centuries by natives of western South America, and as an antidote to high altitude lassitude and dysentery.

For homeopathic preparation the leaves are tinctured and processed. This remedy today is particularly suited to treating the elderly who suffer shortness of breath. It is used by mountaineers for the same symptoms. And it is also useful for related respiratory complaints such as asthma and angina.

Remedies Made from Healing or Holy Waters

Carlsbad Aqua

Carlsbad aqua comes from the waters of the Sprudel and Muhlbrudden Springs in Carlsbad, Germany. Clarke, a famous homeopath, studied the historical use of this this famous spa water known for its action on the liver and for its use in the treatment of obesity, diabetes, and gout. He found that the water has high concentrations of sulfites, bicarbonates and chlorides, and that it is extremely rich in minerals. In homeopathic potencies it is useful in treating a weakness of the organs, for constipation, for heat flashes throughout the body and the tendency to take cold.

Aqua Marina

Aqua marina is potentized seawater, taken from clean seawater miles from shore and at a great depth below the surface. It is a great blood purifier and vitalizer, excellent in the treatment of diseases of the skin, kidneys, and intestines. It suits patients who are hypersensitive, have lung problems, and whose symptoms are worse at the seaside. It is also frequently effective with thyroid disorders. Homeopathically prepared Aqua marina is also useful in many cases of seasickness.

Skookum Chuck

Skookum chuck is a homeopathic preparation of water from Medical Lake near Spokane, Washington, which is a well-known healing site of Native peoples in the region. The homeopathic is prepared from dried salt from the waters in the lake. Local tribes in fact held the waters in such reverence that the lands around the lake were referred as "Sahala Lyee Illihe," or "Sacred Grounds," and no tribe traveling to or from the sacred waters was ever harassed by their enemies.

Homeopathically, skookum chuck has proved itself in the treatment of serious eczemas, rheumatism, and tumors, both benign and malignant.

The Future and Past of Homeopathy

Many of these extraordinary homeopathic medicines have been around for a long time. The modern homeopathic pharmacy pursues medicines used historically, stepping in to confirm the observations of traditional healers, and to explore and develop their medicines' potential for modern use.

There is currently considerable homeopathic development going on through research and proving groups around the world, led by dedicated, experienced homeopaths and homeopathic pharmacists looking to recover and discover more remedies. Of particular interest to those pursuing magical themes in medicine, alchemical texts are leading some homeopaths to make remedies of precious metals used in the process of magical transformation. Some of those are: gold, or homeopathic aurum, silver, or argentum, and mercury, or mercurius. Furthermore, sol, or homeopathic sunlight, is being used now to treat health conditions aggravated by exposure to sun such as skin cancer and violent acute headaches.

The homeopathic pharmacy makes for fascinating reading, and provides considerable information on the mental and emotional effects of exposure to common substances, as well as the side-effects of many popular medications used for physical ailments. Work by Clarke, Boericke, Phatak, and Murphy reveals such gems of homeopathic magic as: amphisbena or lizard jaw, apis (as mentioned above), blatta americana and orientale (American and oriental cockroach, used to treat asthma), bufo (toad poison), buthus australis (scorpion venom), castoreum (secretions from the preputial sacs of beavers), and castor equi (horse "thumbnails;" that is to say, extract from the small, oblong horn that grows on the inner side of the leg of the horse just above the fetlock, which is excellent for treating cracked or ulcerated nipples).

In the end, is it fair to connect magic and homeopathy? In doing so are we damaging the position of homeopathy in the critical eyes of modern medicine? Or are we allowing homeopathic medicine to act as a needed window between differing world views that are instinctively, of necessity, drawing closer together after a great deal of time spent apart.

Further clouding the issue is the fact that a definition of what what is magic and what is not is difficult to ascertain, as one's own beliefs are seldom if ever connected with magical practices, while those of other people who differ are often considered to be magic, superstition, witchcraft, and so on. This sense of perjoration has not helped us keep clear where science and magic begin and end.

Upon closing, for those of you who may need to return to more conservative ground if only for a moment, consider this: homeopathic remedies made from conventional medications such as cortisone, morphine and codeine are proving useful in treating illnesses while avoiding the more disturbing side-effects that accompany these medications. Morphine, derived from opium, is a valuable pain killer following traumatic surgery, but brings with its numbing gift a number of disturbing effects, including a potential for post surgical psychosis. For some, particularly elderly patients, the condition may never abates. Under certain conditions, post surgical depression can be relieved with homeopathic application of morphine in several highly diluted homeopathic potencies. Who care then what we call it—magic, science, or whatever—as long as the treatment is effective.

In Praise of Fat

By Leeda Alleyn Pacotti

The Truth about Obesity

If the truth be told, when we were children many of us teased the fat boy on the bus or the chubby girl in the classroom. Of course, these children hid away from our taunts in the library or science lab, found inward acceptance, and laid the foundations for very bright futures as doctors, lawyers, and computer-whizzes. And we thought we were so clever—at least, until we were older, when we became scornful over our own increasing midlines.

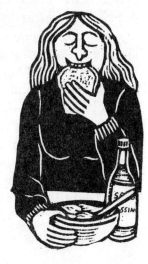

Unfortunately, as adults, we aren't as resilient as those youthful targets of our teasing. We also have learned a lot—that fat was bad, as every dispassionate professional and every smug advertisers took every opportunity to remind us. We looked at endless-magazine articles and health reports warning us about fat.

In the end, we soon found ourselves on a road of oblivion, chasing a chimera of thinness, frightened that we'd succumb to a hideous lifestyle called obesity. Yet, no matter how much we tried to be thin, we couldn't lose our desire for lusciously smooth, comfortingly textured fat. We couldn't avoid the temptation of food—luscious, delicious, endless food, food, food.

Wonderful Fat

Though every person should be concerned about their health as they grow older, there are some basic misconceptions about our dietary needs. For instance, contrary to modern belief, the body requires fat—though certainly, it doesn't need every kind of fat. Fat accumulation in the body, called adipose tissue, creates heat and energy when burned, provides insulation and a cushion between the skin and skeletal masses, sheathes miles of nerves, and participates in most reactions of the body, acting as a carrier of the fat-soluble vitamins A and E and essential fatty acids.

In fact, consumption of essential fatty acids, or EFAs, is an important reason why we must have certain fats in our regular diet. EFAs, sometimes also called vitamin F or polyunsaturates, are not manufactured by the body and can only be found in foods. These important building blocks of nutrition produce very desirable effects in the body. Hair and skin improve. Blood pressure reduces, as do the levels of cholesterol and triglycerides in the blood. Systemic illnesses, such as candidiasis, cardiovascular disease, eczema, and psoriasis, can be allayed through the introduction of EFAs in the diet. High concentrations of EFAs build in the brain, which uses these fat components to aid the neural impulses to other parts of the body. Furthermore, EFAs are required by every living cell to rebuild itself.

Without sufficient EFAs in the body, a person experiences an inability to learn or recall stored information. Skin also dries and flakes, as cellular integrity is compromised. Because cells have greater difficulty reproducing themselves, metabolic and organic functions of all types start to malfunction.

EFAs fall into two categories, called omega-3 and omega-6, designated by their molecular chaining. Omega-3 oils are found predominately in fresh deep water fish, fish oil, and some vegetable oils. Omega-6 oils are exclusively derived from vegetable oils. A few EFAs have become well known. Eicosapentanoic acid, or EPA, and dodecahexanoic acid, or DHA, are part of the omega-3 group; these EFAs benefit the body by lowering blood pressure and regulating cholesterol levels. DHA is prevalent in mother's milk and assists eye and brain development in children. Gamma linoleic acid, or GLA, is a triple unsaturated fat within the omega-6 group; it relieves neural stresses.

The polyunsaturated oils, rich in EFAs, are liquid at room temperature. To derive their benefits, these oils must be consumed cold or raw, because heating destroys any EFAs present. Generally, the daily requirement of EFAs for the body is approximately 10 to 20 percent of the total caloric consumption. The highest presences of omega-3 EFAs are found in cod liver oil, as well as canola oil, flaxseed oil, and walnut oil. Salmon, mackerel, herring, and sardines are also very high in omega-3 fats. Omega-6 EFAs are found abundantly in borage, grape seed, primrose, sesame, soybean, linseed, and safflower oils. Foods rich in omega-6 fats include raw nuts, seeds, legume vegetables, and wheat germ.

Another fat group, which helps the body, are mono-unsaturated fats, of which olive oil is the most well known. These fats are also clear liquid at room temperature, but become cloudy when refrigerated. Oleic acid is the primary EFA present in olive oil. This fatty acid helps in transporting good cholesterol in the blood stream and protects arterial walls from plaque build-up.

Damaging Fat

Of course, there are harmful fats. These outlaws receive regular recognition in commercials and health reports. Bad fat, known as saturated fats, given their high molecular stability, are hard for the human body to digest or break down chemically.

Saturated fats, which remain solid at room temperature, include animal fats, cream, butter, and hard vegetable fats such as coconut and palm oil. These fats, because they tend to accumulate in the blood stream, are the cause of increased cholesterol levels and high blood pressure. Saturated fats also are precursors of a hormone-like substance that creates inflammatory effects, sometimes resulting in eczema or arthritis. In all, saturated fats are very harmful when introduced into the digestive system.

A Scrutiny of Obesity

As already mentioned, our bodies store fat for later production of energy. As the human body evolved over time, scarcities of food and infrequent eating forced the body to develop efficient storage sites that would not interfere with the need for quick physical movements for hunting and migration. Fat storage took up less space in the body and produced more energy, compared to stored volumes of other foods.

While fats from leafy plants and proteins from fish and meat were readily available, carbohydrate foods from roots and sugary plants required special cultivations or were available only in certain seasons. Had these carbohydrate foods been more prevalent and the human body evolved to store them for energy, the modern adult body would be 225 percent more bulky than it is now. In other words, a modern woman of 5'8", who weighs a trim 150 pounds, would weigh a comely 337 pounds, within the reasoning of carbohydrate storage.

This extreme difference in weight expectation from food ingestion brings us precisely to the problem of obesity, a condition of how the body handles consumed foods. Obesity is not simply being overweight. The condition of obesity occurs when a person weighs 20 percent or more over her or his desirable maximum weight. Using our 5'8" woman, her maximum desirable weight is 155 pounds; she would be considered obese, when her weight is 186 pounds or greater. The sin of gluttony is also not an issue here. Gluttony is a self-willed state of excess, in which the individual simply wants everything, without any concern for the consequences. Obese people do not want to be obese, but they are in a vicious spiral of consequences, which leave them feeling powerless. The concern about obesity in modern life arises from how the individual treats her or his own body through eating. In allopathic medicine, the health condition of obesity generally is recognized as a body with too much fat, although this could be better stated as too much flesh. A premise of orthomolecular nutrition simply considers obesity to be caused by overconsumption of processed carbohydrates rather than by proteins and fats.

Other health traditions, such as Ayurvedic medicine, Chinese herbal medicine, and naturopathy or natural cure, also recognize obesity, roughly using the same weight indicator as allopathy. However, the idea of fat ingestion as the sole agent for obesity is not entertained. In these health approaches, obesity is seen as a condition of excess, stagnation, and toxicity complicated by disruption or diminution of digestive processes. These health approaches view obesity as a result of weakened digestion, which in turn overloads the organs of assimilation and elimination.

From this viewpoint, the digestion process is corrupted first by overeating or continually ingesting more food than the system can reasonably handle. Continuous digestion places a burden on the organs of assimilation, namely the pancreas, liver, and gallbladder, forcing them to diminish their vital stores of nutrients used to break down foods before these enter the small intestine. When undigested foods enter the small intestine, that organ has no ability to absorb nutrients from whole foods. Consequently, nutrients demanded by the organs of assimilation never reach them through the blood, compelling assimilation organs into stagnation or hypoactivity. Further, whole food pieces continue the length of the small intestine into the large intestine where, despite its muscular ability to move shapeless food waste along, it becomes filled with heavy food particles. These food particles absorb any moisture in the large intestine, making them even heavier. The result is constipation, in which bowel wastes accumulate, permitting rancidities and toxicities to pass through the large intestinal wall directly into surrounding tissues.

This overview of digestion and assimilation describes the alternative health viewpoint of obesity as excess (overeating), stagnation (hypoactive organs of assimilation), and toxicity (constipation). In the world, the obese person is observed to emulate lifestyle changes that compare roughly to these descriptions. She or he is excessive in size, stagnate in movement, and sometimes seen to have toxic appearances, such as pimples, boils, rashes, or unhealed sores, as the skin takes over as the primary organ of elimination.

Unfortunately, obesity represents a vicious cycle. Because the individual cannot obtain necessary nutrients of vitamins, minerals, and amino acids from foods, she or he remains hungry, even after eating. More food is eaten, in hopes of physical satisfaction, as organs relay neural messages to the brain that they are starving. The result is frustration for the organs, the entire body, and the emotional psyche of the individual, who now feels helpless to change the situation. Worse yet, an overweight, stagnant, toxic body is a ripe field for infections, microbial invasions, and other systemic disorders.

Ending Obesity

The first step in stopping obesity is to gain personal objectivity. One needs to understand that this body is yours, and you are the only one who can nurture it or give it what it needs to maintain its health. At the same time, however, you should know that you are not without resources to regain your health. Your body sends signals constantly to the brain about what it needs. Paying attention to those signals and satisfying them will put you on the road to setting things right. Objectivity about obesity also means recognizing that an obese condition does not come on overnight. It took some period of time for you to become heavy; it will take some time for you to lose the weight.

After regaining your objectivity about your body, visit your health practitioner. You need an assessment about what your proper weight should be, given your physical type and your age. You will be told if it is unrealistic to expect to meet the weight of your teenage years, if you are a full-grown adult. You will also be given a healthy weight guideline appropriate for your physical build. An expectation to be thin as a reed is inappropriate, when your muscular and skeletal formations indicate strength and power. In these discussions with your health provider, you can also bring up questions about genetic ancestry and what influences it may have on your body. (As a side note, if your genetic ancestry was derived from another region of the world within the last 200 years, consider researching foods and activities that were common to that environment. It is possible that your body needs nutrients from foods that are unavailable in your region).

Before outlining any overall approach to changing your obese condition, consider asking your health practitioner to place you on a monitored fasting program. Fasting will cause some hunger and fatigue—physical sensations that already accompany obesity. However, fasting has one important consequence: It gives your organs of digestion, assimilation, and elimination a much-needed rest and recuperation. If your health provider approves a fasting program, expect that you will be allowed to pursue it for no more than five days. Fortunately, a monitored fast can be repeated after about three to six months.

Next, expect to alter your dietary intake. As mentioned before, most obesity is caused by eating too many carbohydrates. Most of these are found in refined, boxed, or prepared foods. The biggest culprits are refined grains, such as white flour, refined sugar, and table salt. None of these ingredients have nutritive value, and they help bring on the vicious food cycle—

the more you eat them, the more you crave them. Carbohydrates generally increase body bulk and do not produce energy or build muscle. In a refined state, they are deficient in vitamins and minerals, which various organs need to create enzymes and hormones to keep the body functioning in optimal condition. Most likely, your health provider will ask you to remove cakes, pies, ice cream, breads, muffins, waffles, pancakes, and other grain foods from your diet for some interval of time. You will also be directed to eat more fruits and vegetables, salads, and digestible fats. Overall, your food portions will decrease.

As your excesses from carbohydrates are diminished, your health provider will suggest ways to end physical stagnancy. Movement is the opposite of stagnation. What movements are best for you will change over the time of your weight reduction. In the beginning, you will be asked to take walks. Walking is a full-body workout and excellent for cardiovascular health. At first, you may not be able to go far, but distance will increase as you gain muscle strength and stamina. You will also be asked to limber up. Stretching and yoga exercises will help you reacquaint with your body's natural movements and tone specific muscle groups. Gung-ho exercise programs, high-level aerobics, and body-building are not specifically necessary as you begin to lose weight. Rather, if you feel a need to return to a more vigorous lifestyle, consider taking up activities you enjoyed as a child or teenager. Biking, swimming, dancing, track and field, and team sports have all reentered adult and elderly physical life. Or, you might consider tackling a sport or activity you had always wanted to try, but felt unable to accomplish. The key in adding movement and exercise to your life is doing what you enjoy, especially anything that fulfills mental pictures you have about yourself.

Some Additional (Herbal) Support

As you make determinations to change your physical body, you might consider herbal supplements to help your digestion. A tea from fennel seed stimulates digestion and prevents accumulations of fat. If you experience a weight gain after a fasting program, astragalus, or yellow vetch, strengthens the digestion and raises metabolism. It also feeds and tones the spleen, an organ of assimilation, and provides a light diuretic effect for the kidneys, another organ of elimination. Discuss these herbs with your health provider, who may have suggestions for other herbal remedies tailored for your physical needs.

Emotional considerations cannot be minimized during weight changes. You may experience shifts between joy and exhilaration over your weight reduction, as well as sadness or depression if you become confused about your new world and new activities. Flower remedies act on emotional well-being. Both English and North American remedies, are available over the counter, complete with directions about how to use them. At the point of purchase, you will find questionnaires and other literature in helping you select a remedy for the emotion you experience. In the event your choice is incorrect, the remedy will simply have no effect on your emotional state. And fortunately, you cannot overdose with flower remedies, which are normally taken in dilution. They can also be modified in dosage for alcohol-sensitive persons. For those who feel powerless to change an obese condition, consider the flower remedy, blackberry. For depression over fulfilling weight expectations, elm is helpful. If the depression arises from physical exhaustion during rapid changes in weight, try olive. Grief sometimes arises from weight loss, because you may not be able to imagine a new future or you are stuck in a sense of failure about the past. Honeysuckle will help you let go of the past, and bring you to a sense of the present. Sagebrush creates acceptance of pain and emptiness, when you feel a sense of loss over your previous lifestyle. If you suppressed feelings of isolation because of your obesity or forced yourself to forfeit desired relationships or activities, yerba santa helps release internalized sadness, especially if those feelings cause pains in the heart region or chest.

You can also purchase homeopathic remedies, in low potencies, over the counter. These are usually available in different strengths, do not require a doctor's supervision, and come with directions for use. Most people who suffer obese conditions have a depletion of the mineral sulfur, which is directly involved in metabolizing fats. A 1x or 6x potency of sulfur will replenish this mineral in the body. However, if you find you have an intolerance for dairy products, forego this remedy, until you feel comfortable eating them again.

. Misunderstandings about fat and the body have spawned crazes of diets and fads for most of the 20th Century. As we
· begin a new era, knowledge about our bodies' nutrition, especially the need for energizing fat, becomes even more critical, given recent traditions of sedentary lifestyle. Knowing we can alter the present condition of our bodies and release the vicious cycle of obesity allows us to regain joy for life and living. With new bodies and minds, we can resurrect our hopes for a good life and build our world anew.

Resisting Environmental Sensitivities

⇒ By Leeda Alleyn Pacotti ⇐

ittle Sally walks into the living room, scratching her arms and neck, complaining with every movement even though she's had her bath and appears fresh as a daisy. In the nursery, six-month-old Mikey has every indication of colic—his protruding abdomen sends him into squalling fits—but nothing seems to help. Meanwhile, after a long day of yardwork in preparation for autumn, Dad lounges in front of the television, coughing loudly as the furnace blower begins its seasonal kick-in. Finishing the clean-up after dinner, Mom sits down at the table with a cup of instant hot cocoa. She listens to the family's complaints and wonders in the back of her mind if she'll ever fit a size 12 again. Amazingly, this scenario of family night has become commonplace in households around the world. Everyone seems to be ill or on the verge of it.

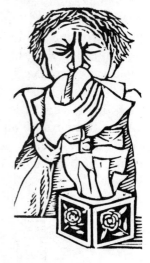

In comparison, most families fifty years ago enjoyed a robust, lively health. A mother of the 1940's or 1950's would have been aghast to find herself and all family members ill. In the last twenty years or so, sensitivities and allergies to foods of all kinds have been on the rise. Sensitivities and allergies cause inappropriate responses from the body's immune system to substances normally not considered harmful. These conditions are so subtle and pervasive that we scarcely notice how common it has become; nearly every family has at least one member who deals with these problems.

With this in mind, doctors and other health practitioners have begun to raise important questions. Has our society become unhealthy beyond a point of return? Are we witnessing an escalating health problem that has doomed us to a life of constant illness and curtailed life-expectancy?

The Major Causes of Sensitivities

In modern life, we move about in surprisingly small environments. Though we live with an illusion of high activity—due to the stressfully fast pace of our world—we forget that we are tied to one place or another for longer periods of time than was true for our forebearers.

Furthermore, because of the demands to meet responsibilities and deadlines and remain a participant in a variety of social activities, we spend minimal attention on personal health. We develop routines, which allow us mental satisfaction of fulfilling conscious demands, but these routines quickly become unconsciously rot activities that cut into the possible diversity of our activities. In fact, unconscious habit is the primary cause of most of our modern sensitivities. With repetition in habit or lifestyle, we continuously expose ourselves to the same conditions of environment, lifestyle, or diet. That is to say, we don't have to think about the changing needs of our bodies as they alter through a lifetime. We begin to think there is one specific answer or product or method, that will keep us safe and secure or healthy and filled with well-being. We forget that remaining in an unhealthy environment for long periods, eating the same foods continually, or using the same products over and over causes our bodies to register certain conditions, foods, or chemicals as inimical to continued good health.

This happens because in general, the body's immune system works by remaining ever-vigilant for invasion by harmful substances. Any invading organism, whether from a cut or wound or from repetitive introduction into the body, must be countered and neutralized by immune defenses. The continual response of the immune system to repeated or prolonged stimulation from perceived harmful substances most often appears in the form of sensitivities or allergic responses.

Sneezing, skin rashes and hives, labored breathing, cold symptoms, flu symptoms, and fevers manifest as the most common allergic responses. But other mechanisms, less identifiable as immune response, also accompany the process. Continual fatigue, muscle soreness, abdominal queasiness or distension, headaches, and backaches can be the result of the operations of the immune system. Without necessary rest, the body can inhibit the immune system, causing allergic stimulants to gain influence over other systems and organs. Then, as such stimulations continue, the body has no choice but to become sicker and more open to other illnesses or infections, as the defensive abilities of the immune system are overwhelmed.

How We Make Ourselves Sick

Surprisingly, except for a congenitally malfunctioning body, most of us are in control of exposure or ingestion of substances which do our bodies harm. Any sense that you have no control or power over the situation is untrue.

In actuality, most of the physical assaults we face daily come from choices we have made without thoroughly examining all consequences or factors involved. For example, an already ill or severely allergic person will often justify remaining in a detrimental situation or habit, even when it is clear that situation or habit intensifies into illness. Furthermore, often a lack of awareness can compound physical conditions which have begun to hamper or harm physical well-being. Often, we suspect we are becoming ill or have a physical condition which is worsening, but we simply refuse to examine our surroundings or lifestyle to discover any underlying cause.

The primary reason for refused awareness about the body's true condition lies in the prevalent idea that illness is weakness, rather than the body's attempt to return itself to good health. Lack of awareness and refused awareness are excellent examples of mind over matter. We avoid knowing we have physical problems, because we don't want to incur the stigma of weakness. We then make choices in lifestyle which perpetuate or aggravate those problems. Later, when we are completely ill or have to forfeit preferred activities, we wonder how we got here.

What seems a vicious cycle of thinking and action can easily be changed, often without resorting to expensive health specialists or neutralizing medications. Because most sensitivities recur almost daily, we are intimately involved with them. A change of perspective to a thorough questioning and examination of lifestyle and environment yields interesting answers that can completely reverse all states of illness.

Three major categories comprise the areas of daily repetitions which cause the body to become sensitized. These are activities, exposures, and dietary improprieties.

Activities

Activities, which sensitize the body's defenses, include specific motions are repeated for several hours on a daily basis. These motions can occur in confined work spaces, and include such actions as continual typing, assembly line work, and heavy lifting. The overall effect from these repetitions wears down the muscles involved because they do not have adequate rest from tasks or an adequate period to integrate nutrients and become replenished. Consequently, the body experiences muscle fatigue and weakness in one area that is constantly being degenerated by the continued activity. Degenerated muscles then become open to infection from normally noninvasive microbial life.

Exposures

Each day, each of us is exposed to potentially harmful substances in our immediate environment. Though we often take precautions to limit the exposure and nullify any continued effects of substances we know to be harmful, we cannot catch everything, and exposures to deleterious substances do occur on a regular and daily basis. In this category fall exposures to domestic chemicals and air pollutants. Such exposures primarily affect the skin through contact and lungs through respiration. A secondary effect of exposure through the lungs is a loss of proper oxygen, necessary for nourishing all tissues throughout the body. Rashes and hive reactions on the skin indicate that the immune defense system has mobilized and begun fighting an absorption, which prevents the skin from performing its function as an eliminative organ. Labored breathing or a sense of general fatigue from a low oxygen content in the body is a clue that the immune system, while working, may be overwhelmed, especially because the entire body is affected.

Dietary Improprieties

Perhaps, the most insidious sensitivities arise from dietary improprieties whic cause the body to be malnourished. Because we have a large selection of foods at our disposal today, most of us believe we cannot be malnourished. However, limited diets, such as meat only or fruit only, fail to give the body a full complement of vitamins, minerals, amino acids, and other nutrients necessary for nourishing specific physical systems, organs, and glands. Ingestion of a high percentage of prepared foods, rather than fresh foods, eventually results in undernourishment, because these preparations contain chemical preservatives with no nutritional value that disrupt digestion and gradually sensitize the digestive system.

Malnutrition and the failure to maintain physical health also result from repetitive diets, in which a specific food is eaten at least daily or at every meal. Repetitive eating is addictive eating; the mind and emotions are satisfied but the body is not. Common foods that can be included in an addictive diet include cow's milk, caffeine drinks, alcohol, chocolate, and wheat products.

Poor eating habits can result even when people think they are maintaining a good dietary pattern. For intance, incorrect cooking methods can rob foods of valuable nutrients. Certain types of cooking utensils not only displace nutrients necessary for good health, but also leave toxic chemical traces in the body. As an example, aluminum cookware binds its metal to most foods, particularly those with any amount of acidity. When the food is ingested, the body absorbs the aluminum, which is one of the few metals in chemical compound that can pass the blood-brain barrier and built up in the brain. Symptoms of aluminum toxicity are very similar to those of Alzheimer's Disease, and research has shown there is a connection between high concentrations of aluminum in the brain and the incidence of Alzheimer's.

Eventually, poor eating affects the entire body because the digestive system uses all available enzymes and naturally occurring chemical compounds to break down one principal food or food group. Other foods go undigested, and their nutrients are eliminated as waste. Ultimately, because necessary nutrients do not enter the blood stream to nourish digestive organs, the digestive system fails, allowing undigested food particles to enter the blood stream. An already overburdened immune system is triggered into action to attack these food particles and protect the blood. Unfortunately, at this point, the entire body is too physically depressed to defend itself in part or in entirety. The compound situation of dietary improprieties, an undernourished body, and an overburdened immune system leave the body open to attack, especially from viruses, which further breaks down the immune system.

Four-fold Plan to Recapture Good Health

As potentially disastrous as sensitizing conditions may sound, each of us can take steps to control and eventually eliminate their effects. Simply stated, you have to consider every one of your habits—whether in lifestyle or environment—a candidate for change. An old health joke drives home the point: "Does it hurt when you do this? Then stop doing it!"

The first step is a critical examination of your lifestyle. Look objectively at your activities, your home and workplace, and your eating habits. How do you labor with your physical body? Does your work at home or in the workplace involve a physical task or posture that you must repeat or maintain for long hours without interruption? How is your breathing affected? Are you regularly exposed to air pollutants such as smoke or smog? Are your lungs assaulted by mold, animal dander, or chemical fumes? What comes in contact with your skin? Do you use chemical detergents regularly to clean yourself? What are you eating? Are you undereating, failing to give your body enough nutrition? Do you tend to eat only one food group or particular type of food? Does your diet consist of many prepared foods or do you eat primarily at restaurants that use prepared foods almost exclusively?

The second step is to confront your conscious mind, especially its justifications for perpetuating habits that create physical sensitivities. Discovering your justifications requires that you confront them. This particular step in the process to return to good health may be very difficult for some people, even more difficult than implementing solutions. Your reasons for perpetuating habits or activities that are deleterious to your health may carry a strong attraction to perpetuate them. Beware of such attractions. Often, you will overemphasize the good results of your choices, without considering what ills also attend them. For instance, a person who lives in a smoggy metropolitan area may justify that a high-income and employee benefits will secure the future. However, no thought is given to how much of that income or those benefits are spent on doctor's visits, medications, or a developing health problem that may result in a chronic condition for the rest of your life. Another individual who has found solace in the calming effects of ice cream may be loathe to give up or curtail its consumption. The idea of becoming calm outweighs obtaining adequate nutrients that would ordinarily nourish the nervous system and neutralize the affecting stress.

After confronting your justifications, the third step is making decisions to alter your habits. It is one thing to know you are abusing your body; it is another thing to stop; this is especially true when correcting addictive food habits. When the body has come to expect the effect of eating a particular type of food, it rebels when that food is removed. Physical symptoms such as headaches, nausea, or other digestive irregularities may ensue, making you seek relief by returning to the demanded food. Determination is the key here. The knowledge that you have been harming yourself may not be enough; you must keep in mind always that you are enslaving your body with ill health from which it might never recover without necessary changes.

The fourth step involves implementing solutions. None of these solutions represents a dead-end. That is, you must tell yourself you won't really be giving up anything. What you will do is make substitutions. You will continue to have a home, even if you change residence. You will continue to work, although you may have a different pursuit. You will still use cleaning supplies and personal hygiene products; however, you will find those which are more physically friendly to your body and skin. You will still eat, but the range of foods will broaden, eventually creating more appealing combinations. In fact, your body will begin to hunger for foods you had forgotten you once enjoyed.

Solving the Problems of Environmental Sensitivities

After diagnosing, examining, and deciding to alter the ills of your activities, environments, and dietary habits, the practical takes over. Most of us have been inundated with advertising hype, telling us which products will do us good, keep us clean, keep us healthy, and keep us fit. Beneath the hype, though, are the undisclosed effects, which we encounter after prolonged use. Because we have been conditioned to believe advertising, we fail to recognize or remember there are products that can benefit us more than the more hyped product.

Don't be swayed by ideas that mainstream products and prepared foods are more cost-effective in the long-run. Such claims don't include how costly medical visits and medications can be when the body has become run down. As well, most health-conscious cleaning and hygiene products come in concentrated forms, which make them at least equivalent in cost and usually less expensive than their chemical counterparts. The following discussions offer some suggestions for modifications and changes you can make without going to great expense. With a little research on your own, you will find activities and products which suit your personal preferences.

Repetitive Work Routines

The best way to avoid repetitive work routines and postures is to change employment. Change gives you an opportunity to try a different career and different activities; however, if you are dedicated to your career path, you will need to adopt a movement program that counters repetitive physical movement. Such programs are easy to create, even without resorting to expensive health spas or exercise gymnasiums. Persons, who self-impose physical restrictions or remain at chores overly long, need to review their thinking about relaxation and breaks and come to an understanding of the value of taking a rest. For instance, when limited to a confined space a daily walk, with an increased heart rate for twenty minutes, not only invigorates the entire body, but is excellent for stimulating digestion and releasing toxins through the skin. Individuals, who experience limited hard exertion benefit from slow stretching exercises which relieve

cramped muscles. A half-hour program of counteractive movement is ample to keep the body in tone.

Polluted environments

Individuals who work in pollution and waste clean-up, of course
need to know and understand what regulations are in effect to
protect their health while on the job. For those who reside in
areas of air pollution or near toxic sites, the best remedy is to
move to a clean area. However, while making such a change,
supplements of vitamin B-15 help open the tubules in the lungs,
permitting more oxygen to be accepted during inhalation. Lungs
may also need cleaning. Borage tea, steeped by cold infusion (the
cut herb left overnight in cold water) helps the lungs expel particulate matter. Expect coughing and expectoration of dirty
mucus from the lungs.

Desert sensitivities

Residents in desert areas experience a loss of nutrients through
sweating and dehydration. Usually, allergic reactions to the
environment begin to show about one year after continued residence. In particular, these are stimulated or aggravated during
pollination seasons of trees, weeds, and other indigenous plant
life. Most noticeably, residents exhibit sneezing fits, aggravated
from dry nasal passages, and breathing difficulties, stemming
from dry bronchials. Both are consequences of a low-humidity
atmosphere. To maintain body moisture, desert dwellers need to
consume more salad vegetables than residents of other areas.
The sodium content of these vegetables helps the body retain
moisture. To lessen the impact of pollen sensitivity, residents
benefit from a tablespoon of locally gathered bee pollen, eaten
daily. Because the bee pollen contains minute amounts of plant
pollens, the body becomes desensitized to seasonal pollen
counts. To protect the inner nose, a solution of one part vegetable glycerine to one part spring or distilled water swabbed
inside the nostrils each morning and, if necessary, before bed-
time, keeps the nasal membranes moist and pliant. Inhaling

steam from a bath or a vaporizer will rehydrate dry bronchial tubes. A lotion made from equal parts of vegetable glycerine and aloe vera gel soothes and protects exposed skin from the drying effects of sun and hot winds.

Household chemicals

Most of the products we use around the house are touted as exemplary cleaners. However, the chemicals in them have a vicious effect on the lungs and skin. In reality, natural products, which have little or no effect on the lungs and skin, work just as well as chemical cleaners, if not better at times. In keeping your home clean, consider the following changes. For dishes and clothing, a pine oil compounded into a castile soap base is excellent for cleaning and dissolving grease and oils. In laundry, one-quarter cup of baking soda per washing load eliminates odors from clothing. When added to hot water, pine resin releases a nice scent, deodorizing surrounding air. White vinegar is excellent for neutralizing smells, especially carpet stains by animals; this makes an excellent final rinse on floors. White vinegar, allowed to stand at least one-half hour in the toilet bowl, dissolves lime deposits, which are easily loosened with a bowl brush. Household bleach absolutely sanitizes the toilet bowl; remember to rinse your hands with cold water, if you accidentally splash bleach on your skin. Tung nut oil or olive oil absorb deeply into natural woods, bringing out rich grain and tones. To keep wood furniture in top condition, softened or melted beeswax will protect any finish.

Personal Hygiene

Many beauty products contain petroleum-based chemicals. In areas with high particulate matter from traffic congestion, these products attract the particulate to skin and hair, causing skin reactions and decreasing hair lustre. Consequently, shampoos and conditioners made from petroleum products require more frequent shampooing, which removes natural emollients from hair. Organic shampoos clean hair well, without attracting a build-up of oil or grime from the air. Castile soap, made with olive oil, also gently cleans hair without stripping natural oils. A regular after-shampoo rinse of juice from one or two lemons, combined with two quarts of chamomile tea for light hair or sage tea for dark hair, restores the pH level, invigorates the scalp, and reduces scalp dryness. Skin also benefits from castile soaps, scented with natural oils from peppermint, lavender, or eucalyptus. For facial cleansing, these soaps, applied with a facial brush, clean deep pores, soothe the skin, and tone the underlying muscular structure. A follow-up astringent of witch hazel, based in an alcohol solution, increases circulation and imparts a healthy glow. For those whose skin is beginning to show signs of wear from the elements, a solution of one part vegetable glycerine with two parts spring or distilled water returns moisture to delicate tissues around the eyes and mouth, plumping the thinner skin and ironing out wrinkles. By keeping the outer lids moist, dryness on the eyeball is reduced. As for other hygienic commercial products, many people have a fascination with presumed body aroma. In most situations, body odors are intensified by laundry detergents. However, some are attributable to ingestion of repetitive foods. As the body attempts to expel certain by-products of digestion, it utilizes the skin, which is an eliminative organ. Individuals who feel the need for a deodorant can consider switching to a product that contains no aluminum, which can be absorbed directly through the skin and into the bloodstream.

Dietary Changes

Because food is distributed throughout the body faster than contact chemicals, systemic sensitivities appear slowly and become more pronounced over time. A two-step analysis of you diet will uncover hidden food allergies. First, keep a four-week diary of everything eaten without giving much thought to the exact types of foods. An honest record is best. While this diary is kept, note also any reactions that occur during or after eating. These reactions will usually show within one hour and may appear as nasal congestion, coughing, wheezing, itching, headache, increased heart rate, or a sense of fatigue. After the four weeks are up, your next step is to make a critical review of the diary. Make a special note of physical reactions. Observe which foods were eaten before those reactions. Note any foods which were eaten four or more times in any one week. These two sets of foods are your list for suspected food sensitivities or allergies. Next, omit all these suspected foods from your diet for thirty days. Eliminating them gives your digestive tract and your entire body an opportunity to rest and replenish any depleted nutrients. After the thirty-day period, introduce each of the suspected foods one day at a time. If you note any reaction to a reintroduced food, immediately eliminate it from your diet. Go through the entire suspect list, then wait two months have passed. At the end of two months, try a small amount of the suspect food again. If you still have a reaction, eliminate that food permanently from your diet.

Other Food Changes

As mentioned before, poor cooking habits can undermine a good nutrition. Overcooking foods destroys valuable nutrients. Rather than preparing vegetables or fruits through boiling or browning, try eating them raw. If raw foods are disagreeable, steam vegetables and fruit or stir-fry them to a light tenderness in an iron wok. Foods with any kind of burn, such as burned toast or bread or flame-cooked meats, create substance called heterocyclic aromatic amines, which, under laboratory conditions, have been shown to be a precursor of cancer. Meats are particularly susceptible for developing carcinogenic compounds. To understand the seriousness of the problem of burned food, one-half gram of ingested burned food has a carcinogenic volume equivalent to inhaled smoke from two packs, or forty cigarettes.

Toxicity from improper cooking utensils wreaks a two-fold disaster on the body. Besides causing a chemical interaction with food, permitting toxicities to enter the body, valuable nutrients are displaced or are converted to an unusable compound.

Aluminum cookware and storage containers produce a substance in foods that neutralizes digestive juices in the body; this neutralization can lead to ulcers throughout the digestive system. Aluminum in the body has an affinity for the brain and nervous system, where it tends to accumulate. The results are neural disorders and symptoms resembling Alzheimer's Disease.

Cookware with enamel coatings often contains cadmium, a toxic trace mineral, which accumulates most often in the liver and kidneys and replaces essential zinc. Cadmium can also enter the body from first or second-hand cigarette smoke. This toxicity weakens the immune system, can lead to kidney disease, and seriously damage the liver.

Nonstick coatings on cooking utensils are made from toxic chemicals. During cooking, these chemicals interact with foods. When food is removed from the pans, possible flecks of the coating can end up in food servings.

Plastic containers for food and beverage storage also carry a level of toxicity, because plastic will interact with food. Consequently, chemical compounds from plastic, which are petroleum based, will accumulate in the body, but not be absorbed.

All types of cookware and storage containers, that can produce toxicity, need to be removed once and for all from your kitchen. Replace them with glass or Corning ware, which do not interact with food during heat processes. Stainless steel or iron cookware are acceptable, because they contain iron, which is not toxic. Your physical health is a valuable asset, meant to sustain you for a lifetime. Making changes to preserve its integrity against the onslaughts of activities, environments, and improper diet not only keeps you in a state of balanced well-being, but gives you robust energy to tackle exciting challenges. Returning to or maintaining good health is not a chore or career, it's simply your choice.

Herbs
for
Beauty

Creating an Herbal Health Spa

❧ By Judy Griffin, Ph.D. ❧

*Y*ou can create a personal home spa to nurture your skin and heal your psyche. The regular use of an herbal home spa will have numerous beneficial effects. It will give you radiant skin and turn a tedious day into an extraordinary experience. And in fact, your personal spa can be superior to that of the finest European health spas at only a fraction of the price.

The herbs you use in your herbal health spa should be organically produced and free from all damaging pesticides or chemical fertilizers. Essential oils must also be steam-distilled and separated without chemical treatment. Choose the finest ingredients to restore the beauty inherent in your skin. You should strive to create a regular routine to include simple massage techniques to

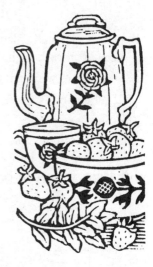

alleviate tension and stress. The following recipes will cast a healing environment from your head down to your toes.

Scalp Shampoo and Conditioner

Here's a shampoo that will clean the scalp and encourage healthy hair growth.

Daily Shampoo Formula

4 tablespoons liquid castile soap

1 teaspoon fresh avocado cold-pressed oil

4 drops peppermint essential oil

1 cup water

4 tablespoons fresh gotu kola, minced, or horsetail

1 teaspoon willow bark, ground

Combine castile soap, oil, and essential oil. Set aside. Boil water. Remove from heat. Add gotu kola and willow bark. Cover and steep 30 minutes. Strain liquid through cheesecloth. Allow to cool and combine with liquid castile mixture. Bottle in a clean plastic container with a spout. Use a dime to quarter size amount daily, scrubbing the scalp vigorously.

Vinegar Rinse

To restore the acid balance of the scalp, use a vinegar herbal rinse in place of store-bought conditioners.

1 cup hot, white vinegar

2 tablespoons fresh, lavender essential oil

Combine vinegar and lavender oil. Cover and allow to infuse 15 minutes. Strain lavender leaves, if used, and massage warm vinegar into scalp and hair after shampoo. Store remaining liquid in a dark glass or plastic container with a tight plastic lid.

Herbal Conditioner

For those who want to treat damaged hair and stimulate new hair growth, use this conditioner once or twice weekly.

 1 cup water

 1 tablespoon fresh rosemary leaves

 1 tablespoon St. John's Wort oil

 1 egg yolk

Bring water to boil. Remove from heat and add rosemary leaves. Cover and allow to steep 10 minutes. Strain. Allow to cool 10 minutes . Stir in St. John's Wort oil. Beat in egg yolk after mixture reaches room tempurature. Apply to scalp and hair, massaging gently for 3 minutes. Rinse with warm water, then repeat with cool water. (Note: you may substiture rosemary water for the essential oil. Make by adding 3 drops of Rosemary essential oil to 1 cup of warm water. Also, to make St John's oil, steep 1 tablespoon of yellow flowers from the Hypericum perforatum plant in full bloom in ½ cup warmed vegetable oil of your choice for 7–21 days until the oil turns deep red. Strain and bottle in a clean glass container.)

Deep Cleaning Facial Steam

Steam the face once or twice weekly to remove blackheads and reduce breakouts.

 1 quart water

 2 drops bergamot

 4 drops geranium

 1 drop lemongrass

 1 drop sage or clary sage

Boil the water. Remove from heat and add essential oils. Create a tent with a clean, fresh bath towel. Allow the vapor to lightly steam the face and open the pores for 5 to 10 minutes. Follow with a cold water rinse and gently pat the face dry.

Rejuvenating Blend for Delicate or Tired Skin

For those with clear skin, use a rejuvenating blend.

- 2 cups very warm water
- 1 drop basil oil
- 3 drops lavender oil
- 1 drop sandlewood oil
- 1 drop palmarosa or rose oil

Combine all ingredients. Soak a clean washcloth in the water. Lie down and apply the fragrant water as a compress on the face. As the water cools, apply a freshly soaked cloth to the face.

Gentle Face Massage

While you are enjoying a facial steam or compress, a light massage will encourage circulation and drainage of excess fluids and cellular waste. Using the lightest pressure, move the fingertips of both hands in an upward motion from the neck to the forehead.

Jojoba Balancing Blend

An excellent balancing blend for sensitive or troubled skin can be prepared with jojoba oil. It is not a true oil, but a liquid wax which easily combines with sebum for penetration. Jojoba will absorb without leaving a greasy feeling to the skin.

- 2 tablespoons pure Jojoba oil
- 2 drops of steam distilled rose oil or 1 drop lavender essential oil or 1 drop carrot seed oil

Combine ingredients; apply to the face and neck in upward strokes.

Eye Massage

To massage around the eyes and brows, carefully make light circles around the eyes with your fingertips. Start at the eyebrows and work toward the nose, using the ring fingers. They have the gentlest touch and do not harm the delicate skin under the eyes.

Puffy Eyecare

For puffy or swollen eyes, use the following recipe to reduce fluid retention. Puffy eyes have many causes: allergies, eyestrain, stress, and overuse of salt. This skin is very delicate and responds best to gentle treatments.

To reduce puffiness, steep 2 teabags of black or oolong tea in 1 cup of very hot water for 5 minutes. Strain and apply warm to closed eyelids for 5 minutes. Remove and follow with a cold rosemary compress.

For the rosemary compress, add 2 teaspoons of fresh rosemary leaves to ½ cup of boiled water. Remove from heat, cover, and allow to steep 15 minutes. Strain. Pulverize 2 ice cubes with the rosemary infusion in a blender. Apply cold with cotton compress bandages cut to fit over the eyes. Lie down and relax for 10 to 15 minutes while nature rejuvenates the eyes.

Sinus Compress

For those who suffer from congested sinus passages, this is an excellent compress to apply after a facial steam and gentle massage. This recipe also tones the pores.

2 cups of very warm water

2 drops dalmation sage

4 drops lemon eucalyptus

Add the essential oils to the warm water. Soak a clean washcloth into the mixture. Lie down and apply the cloth over the sinuses and forehead. Breathe evenly and deeply for 3 to 5 minutes before removing the cloth. Repeat as desired.

Herbal Sinus Remedy

Eucalyptus leaves

Garden sage leaves (Salvia officinalis)

Lemon thyme leaves

Boil 2 cups of water in a saucepan. Remove from heat. Add 2 tablespoons of each herb, singly or in combination as available. Cover and steep for 10 minutes. Strain; allow to cool to a warm room temperature. Soak a clean cloth in the infusion. Lie down comfortably. Apply the cloth over the face. Breathe deeply as the sinuses decongest.

Skin Lightening Treatment

This is a great treatment for brown spots, freckles, darkened knees, and elbows. Be sure to begin with a patch sample on the skin before applying to larger areas. And Avoid eyes and any broken skin.

1 cup buttermilk

5 drops of lemongrass essential oil

2 drops of marigold mint (Tagetes lucida foeniculum) essential oil

Blend ingredients thoroughly and apply to affected areas with a small watercolor brush. Apply successive coats of the mixture before areas dry, keeping the skin moist for twenty minutes. Then allow the skin paint to dry and rinse with warm water.

The treatment can be repeated once daily until skin is lightened. Leftover mixture can be stored in a dark, glass bottle with a screw tight lid in the refrigerator for 1 week. Moisturize before bedtime to reduce dehydration. Use a light touch of moisturizer during the daytime and under makeup.

My Favorite Rose Cream

Here's an old fashion recipe that is very popular at my house. It is an easy, excellent remedy for dry skin and safe for every age.

2 tablespoons fresh rose petals

2 tablespoons rose water, warm

2 tablesppons jojoba oil

2 tablespoons almond oil or coconut oil

8 tablespoons of melted cocoa butter softened over a
double boiler

4 tablespoons vegetable glycerin

Blend the petals and water at high speed. Add the oil mixture and blend for 1 minute. Pour in glass jars, adding 2 drops of distilled rose oil in each jar. Cover with a tightly fitted lid. Store away from heat and light. Apply to dry or chapped skin. (Variations: substitute fresh, lavender flowers and lavender essential oil for rose petals if you prefer a different odor. Blend 2 drops of carrot seed oil in the mixture to alleviate chapped skin.)

Aromatic Herbal Body Wrap

Pamper and restore your entire body with a healing herbal therapy. The following suggestions are comparable to the best spas worldwide.

How to Prepare an Herbal Wrap

Combine 3 cups of fresh herbs of your choice. Add to 8 cups of boiled water. Cover and remove from heat. Steep 30 minutes. Strain and allow to cool just above room temperature, adding 2 cups of Epson salts. Stir to dissolve.

Though you can adapt this recipe to suit your own herbal tastes, you might first choose from the following herbs:

Relaxation: Lavender leaves, Chamomile leaves and flowers,
Sage leaves (Clary or Garden Sage), Orange blossoms,
Jasmine flowers, Lemon Balm leaves (Melissa), scented
Geranium leaves, Rose petals of any fragrant variety.

Stimulating: Mints of any flavor, ground Cinnamon, Cloves, Lemon Grass leaves, Basil leaves and flowers, Marjoram, Oregano, Marigold Mint (Tagetes lucida foeniculum), sliced or ground Ginger root.

Healing antiseptic: Thyme, Eucalyptus leaves, Rosemary, Calendula flowers, Comfrey leaves, Yarrow leaves and flowers.

Healing Antiseptic Recipes

6 Eucalyptus drops

3 White thyme drops

4 Tea Tree drops

2 Pine drops

or

6 Majoram drops

4 Rosemary drops

2 White Thyme drops

2 Lemon Balm drops

1 Amber drop

or

8 Cedarwood drops

3 Myrhh drops

2 Patchouli drops

2 Francinsense drops

Relaxing Blends

8 Lavender drops

3 Clary sage drops

2 Neroli drops

1 Bergamot drops

or

6 Sandlewood drops

4 Rose drops

4 Palmarosa drops

1 Ylang Ylang drop

or

10 Dalmation Sage drops

5 Mandarin Orange or Tangerine peel drops

3 Palmarosa drops

Stimulating Recipes

10 Peppermint drops

2 Oregano drops

4 Marigold Mint drops

1 Grapefruit peel drop

or

6 Lemon Grass drops

4 Basil drops

2 Lime peel drops

6 Spearmint drops

or

6 Cinnamon leaf drops

4 Juniper berries drops

4 Ginger root drops

2 Lime peel drops

What to Do Next

Once you have prepared an aromatic infusion, dress down to your underwear or birthday suit, and find a peaceful setting to relax. Lay a tarp on a comfortable chair. Gather clean cotton strips (from old sheets, for example) and cut them into 2 to 4 inch wide strips, 12 to 24 inches long. Dip into the aromatic herbal infusion. Wring and double wrap each strip around the feet, legs, thighs, hips, midsection, and chest. Then wrap the arms and hands. Tuck the ends under the wrap. Recruit help when available. Make sure the wraps are not too tight. Lie back comfortably in an easy chair and cover your body. Maintain a comfortable body temperature for 30 minutes. Unwrap and pat dry, or follow with a relaxing massage.

Cellulite Wrap for Heavy Areas

Use this blend to increase circulation and reduce adipose tissue. It can be used in areas where you gain weight or as an all over body treatment.

Before wrapping, brush the skin with a dry washcloth or loofah to exfoliate surface skin, increase circulation and lymphatic drainage. Begin with gentle stroking and work into a more vigorous rub as long as you can tolerate it. Work in a circular motion from the lower body to the upper body. Use soft strokes on the breasts and neck.

Herbal Infusion to Reduce Cellulite

Chickweed

Fennel seed, crushed in a mortar and pestle

Dandelion leaves

Chickory leaves

Grapefruit peel, fresh or dried

Peppermint leaves

Oregano leaves

up to ½ cup of powdered Dulse (optional)

In 4 cups of boiled water, add 2 cups of each of the fresh herbs (or 1½ cups of dried herbs). Cover and steep for 30 minutes.

Strain well and wrap as the infusion cools to a comfortable temperature.

Aromatic Essential Oil Cellulite Blend

8 drops geranium oil

6 drops of grapefruit peel oil or lemon grass oil

2 drops of cypress oil

optional: ½ cup seaweed or powdered dulse

    2 drops of juniper berry oil

    2 drops of cinnamon leaf oil or 2 drops of ginger root oil

    2 drops of fennel seed oil or marigold mint oil

Add herbs to 4 cups of hot water. Soak wraps and apply on cellulite. (Note: both seaweed and dulse soften the skin and promote circulation.)

Massage

After an aromatic body wrap, a massage may further increase circulation and remove cellulite and metabolic waste, though it's best to wait a few hours after a wrap before beginning another therapeutic treatment. Enjoy a light lunch or tea break while the body assimilates the value of the wrap.

Massage is a Greek word. It translates " to knead." Physicians of ancient times used massage as a routine form of treatment. Aromatherapy and massage are perhaps the first therapeutic treatments used by healers and physicians. For aromatic massage, stroking movements or effleurage are used. Deep strokes involve the whole hand applying pressure in the direction of the heart to enhance venous flow. The return stroke is superficial, light, slow, and rhythmic, and the hands mold to the body.

If you do not have a professional masseuse available, massage your legs, arms, abdomen, and shoulders with an aromatic blend and promise your body you will make time to follow through with a professional massage in the very near future.

Synergistic Essential Oils

Here are some ideas to combine synergistic essential oils. Blend 3 to 5 oils combining 15 to 20 drops in 2 ounces of a vegetable carrier oil.

Stimulating Essential Oils

Basil, useful for sluggish and congested skin, combines well with Bergamot, Geranium, Hyssop, Lavender, Lemon Grass. Basil opens the sinuses and alleviates headaches.

Bergamot, beneficial for oily and troubled skin, also blends well with cyprus, neroil, lavender, and lemon grass. Bergamot increases photosensitivity. I recommend low doses, 2 to 3 drops, of this citrus flavored aroma with suggested synergistic oils.

Clary Sage benefits inflammed and sensitive skin. Low doses, 3 to 5 drops, blend well with lavender, sandlewood, geranium, frankincense, lemon, lime, and tangerine peel oils. Higher doses are used to reduce anxiety and insomnia.

Eucalyptus is antiseptic, benefitting oily, congested skin. Combine eucalyptus with thyme, lemon grass, pine, marjoram, or basil. The aroma opens the lungs and sinuses quickly letting you know if it is a beneficial aroma for you.

Lemon Grass is a stimulating antiseptic used to cleanse and reduce pores, reduce oil production, and increase lymphatic drainage. Blend lemon grass with eucalyptus, thyme, spearmint, ginger, or lavender, geranium and sandlewood.

Sage benefits congested skin, relieves fluid and sinus congestion and muscle tension. Large doses can reduce lactation. Nursing mothers can use low doses (up to 3 drops.) Please consult a lactation consultant in the event of continued use. Blend sage with lavender, sandlewood, oregano, lemon grass, bergamot, hyssop or marjoram.

Tea tree is an antiseptic used for oily skin and minor wounds. It can be used as well as eucalyptus and thyme, to reduce fungal skin conditions.

Balancing Aromatic Oils

Cypress increases circulation, reduces broken capillaries and inflammed varicose veins and balances oily skin. Blend cypress with juniper berries, pine, Tthyme, sage, lavender and sandlewood.

Geranium cleanses sensitive, inflammed and oily skin. It combines well with rose to enhance mature skin.

Hyssop is an excellent antiseptic for injured, bruised or itchy skin. Blend hyssop with lemon grass, rosemary, sage or lavender. Hyssop is not recommended for epileptics.

Juniper berries reduce dermatitus and seborrhea of the scalp and balances oily skin. Blend juniper with cypress, lavender, and sandlewood.

Lavender balances every skin type, reduces burns, retards warts, relieves anxiety and tension. It can be used alone or combined with citrus flavored oils as an insect repellent, sage or clary sage, and patchouli to relax and sedate the muscles. Lavender and rosemary balance oily and easily irritated skin, while relieveing headaches. Rose attar and lavender blend well for romantic oils that enhance mature skin.

Marigold mint has a fennel flavor with the soothing qualities of marigolds. I use it to reduce brown skin spots, precancerous skin conditions, and melanoma patients (with permission from their physician) in a topical cream. It blends well with citrus oils as an antiseptic to reduce large pores and blackheads. With geranium and lavender, it reduces fluid retention and cellulite. Sandlewood and vetiver or oakmoss can be added as a base note to remove lymphatic impurities.

Peppermint can be used in massage to increase circulation and lymphatic drainage. Stronger blends, 6 to 10 drops in 2 to 3 ounces of carrier oil, sedate the muscles and reduce pain from headaches, arthritis and muscle spasms. Combine with eucalyptus, sage, lavender or oregano to reduce pain. Rosemary and peppermint relieve lymphatic congestion, dandruff and fluid retention.

Rosemary is both cleansing and stimulating to the skin. It can benefit mature and oily skin or hair conditions. Add it to dandruff shampoos or blend with bergamot, citrus, basil and peppermint for a stimulating massage. Lavender blends relieve headaches and mild depression.

Thyme is an excellent antiseptic and decongestant. It blends well with eucalyptus and tea tree to combat flus or colds and decongest the lungs and sinuses. Combined with rosemary it has diuretic and antidepressive effects. Blend it with lemon grass to stimulate hair growth.

Base Notes

Base notes are used to sedate blends, extend penetration, and lengthen aromatic staying power. One or 2 drops are added to hold a blend. It can take 2 to 3 hours for a blend to infuse a carrier oil. When it is necessary to use a blend sooner, add essential oils to a warm carrier oil.

Benzoin is a tree resin commonly known as "friar's balsam." It is a common ingredient in incense. Benzoin combines well with rose, lavender or sandlewood for dry, cracked or irritated skin.

Cedarwood is an ancient aroma used by Egyptians to preserve mummies. It combines well with neroli, citrus oils and rosemary for acne or oily skin and scalp conditions.

Francincense is a rejuvenative resin oil blended with lavender, gerium, myrhh and sandlewood to tone facial skin and sores.

Neroli, Citrus aurantium, is distilled from the flowers of the bitter orange tree. As a base note, it blends well with geranium, clary sage, lavender, and benzoin for dry, cracked skin and broken capillaries.

Oregano—Greek, Italian, Mexican and wild varieties can be used in blends to reduce pain, cellulite, and head lice. Combine it with eucalyptus, peppermint, thyme and sage.

Patchouli reduces fluid retention, nervousness, sores that do not heal and cracked, dry skin. When worn near the face, it opens and drains the sinuses. Combine with rose, neroil, lavender, sandlewood, bergamot, and geranium.

Rose is most healing to all skin types. It benefits sensitive, mature, and inflammed skin. True steam-distilled rose oil is safe for children. It blends well with lavender, geranium, sandlewood, patchouli, sage and clary sage.

Sandlewood, from Mysere in East India, sedates inflammed skin. In India, it is known to calm the mind and open the heart. It benefits dry or inflammed skin combined with lavender, rose, benzoin, frankincense, sage, or neroli.

Lavender Daze

The following recipes will give you a few more ideas on how to blend herbs and essential oils for natural beautycare. When life seems overwhelming or lets you down, leave your troubles behind as you step into a Lavender therapeutic beaty treatment.

Lavender Massage Oil

20 drops of Lavender essential oil

800 IU of vitamin E

2 drops of Peppermint or Sage oil

Choose a rich carrier oil, such as almond, avocado or walnut oil, and add above ingredients to 4 ounces of the carrier oil. Apply warm to clean unbroken skin.

Lavender Bath

If no one is available to pamper you with a massage, draw a tub of warm water and relax in a lavender bath.

To 1 tablespoon cream or honey, add 10 drops of lavender essential oil. Stir into a warm tub of water. Step in, sit back and relax for 15 to 20 minutes as the water gently washes your troubles away.

Lavender Deodorant

If time doesn't allow you the luxury of a relaxing bath or massage, dust your body with a light Lavender powder and spray on this lavender deodorant.

Spray:

2 ounces of Witch Hazel

1 tablespoon Vodka

15 drops of Lavender essential oil

1 drop Lemon Grass oil

2 drops Rosemary oil

Add ingredients to a spray bottle. Shake well before using.

Powder:

1/4 cup Arrowroot

1/4 cup Cornstarch

6 drops of Lavender essential oil

2 tablespoons ground Lavender flowers.

Combine and store in airtight container.

Historical Uses of Lavender

Besides bathing in Lavender water, Romans wore sprigs of lavender in their hair to prevent headaches caused by the sun. Lavender oil was massaged into the skin to prevent nervous ticks. The fragrant water was sniffed or splashed on the skin to prevent fainting. Brides were bathed in lavender water on their wedding day. Nearby in North Africa, lavender blossoms and leaves were added to curry.

Naturally White Tooth Powder

Here's an alternative to expensive, cosmetic bleaching used by American colonists and Native Americans.

Tooth Whitener

Puree 2 large strawberries in a blender. Pour into a bowl. Dip a clean toothbrush into the puree and gently brush onto the teeth. Allow to set 5 minutes and repeat the application of strawberry puree. After 5 minutes, rinse well with the following tooth powder.

1 tablespoon of baking soda

1 teaspoon of cream of tartar

1 drop of tea tree essential oil

1 drop of spearmint, cinnamon or fennel flavoring

Mix well. Sprinkle generously on a toothbrush and brush each tooth gently. Rinse well. Follow with a lemon thyme antiseptic mouthwash and gargle. Steep 1 tablspoon of fresh lemon thyme leaves in 1 cup boiled water, covered, for 10 minutes. Strain.

Allow to cool in the refrigerator up to 3 hours. Use for a mouth-wash and gargle. Refrigerate leftover tea and use within 48 hours.

Nail Nutrients

Apply this salve to ridged and cracked fingernails.

⅓ cup fresh Horsetail

⅓ cup fresh Oatstraw

⅓ cup fresh Comfrey leaves

In a quart pan, bring 1 cup of Avocado oil to simmer. Add herbs, cover, and remove from heat. Steep 30 minutes. Strain to remove all plant material.

Pour the oil into a double boiler. Add 2 tablespoons of grated beeswax. Simmer on low heat until wax melts completely. Remove from heat. Stir, and allow to cool 30 minutes. Add 5 to 6 drops of neroli or lemon grass essential oil. Stir and spoon into ½ ounce containers. Yields 12 jars. (Variation: add 6 drops of lavender and 2 drops of sandlewood essential oil to replace the lemon grass or neroli.)

Herbs in the Bath

～ By Silver Sage ～

Y ou have an important meeting in the morning that
you've been preparing for
for weeks, but suddenly your kids ge
sick and keep you up all night. Or,
perhaps your car is in the shop and
there's not quite enough money to fix
it, but you can't to work to make the
money to get it fixed because you don't
have a car to take you to work. In other
words, there are often times that life
hands you more stress than you can
deal with.

At these times, of course, the que-
siton becomes "What to do, oh, what
to do?" You could jump off a cliff
(which is rather permanent), you could
get drunk (not really a great idea in
general, and a bad example to the kids),
or you could do yourself a favor and
take some time off just for you. In this
case, you lock the bathroom door, play

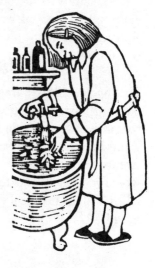

some soothing music, light a few candles, and take a wonderful herbal bath.

Baths have been enjoyed for their pleasure and benefit for centuries. Bathhouses abounded in ancient Rome and Greece. The English and the Russians have been known for their baths at different times in history. Native Americans, too, gathered in warm mineral baths.

Today public baths are usually called "spas," but they accomplish the same thing. The fact remains tha warm water is incredibly soothing and relaxing. In today's break-neck world, soothing herbal baths are probably more necessary than they were even in ancient times.

Herbs have a long history of being life's little helpers. There are herbs that help with all sorts of complaints, and herbs that can be used internally or externally. Sometimes just the fragrance of a certain herb will accomplish enough to make the difference between illness and health. The skin that wraps us all together is the largest organ we have, and it's an organ of excretion. One of the ways that our body cleanses itself is to sweat (excrete) out impurities. Sweat baths have long been used for both their medicinal as well as their religious significance.

So, stands to reason, if you combine the wonderfully therapeutic properties of warm water with the fantastic restorative abilities of herbs, you've got a win-win situation!

The Herbal Bath

Tossing a handful of fragrant herbs and flowers into your tub and bathing with them floating on top of the water may seem a romantic notion, but in fact this method isn't very practical. Who wants to finish a relaxing, romantic or soothing bath and spend twenty minutes picking pieces of herb off of their wet skin! Or worse yet, who wants to call the plumber to clear the drain after all that plant material clogs up the works. Talk about ruining a mood!

Instead, you a good basic method is to tie the herbs up in a piece of cheesecloth or in a muslin bag and hang them from the spout while the water is running. This is much neater, and certainly won't wreck your mental peace and quiet. And you can also use the bag of herbs to scrub your skin. It acts as an exfoliant.

However, probably the best way to get the most out of the herbs is to make a strong infusion of the herbs you've selected and add that to the bath water. This is accomplished by simmering a half-cup of the dried herbs in water for ten to twenty minutes. Roots, coarse stems, or woody herbs should be simmered for twenty to twenty-five minutes. Strain out the herbs and add the liquid to the bath water. Be sure to use a non-metal pot, because metal will often react unfavorably with the herbs.

If you put the herbs into a muslin bag or tie them in a large wash cloth before adding them to the pot, you can still have a great herbal scrubber and a potent infusion to boot! Make sure the herbs have "elbow-room" in the bag or cloth. If they don't have room to expand, the water won't be able to completely saturate the herbs. You'll have dry spots that haven't released their goodness into the water. In effect, you'll have an inferior infusion, and you will have wasted good herbs.

The temperature of the bath water is an important factor, and some attention should be paid to it. Warm water (temps around 97-100 degrees) soothes and relaxes, while cool water (temps around 80 degrees) stimulates. Be wary of very hot baths (temps around 104 degrees or more), this can dehydrate the system, dry the skin, and cause exhaustion. That high a temperature can also be harmful if you have high blood pressure, diabetes, or are pregnant.

There are herbs that are soothing, herbs that invigorate, herbs for healthy, glowing skin, herbs for sore muscles, and herbs to ease a cold. There are herbs to restore your serenity, to calm you, and help you to sleep. Just about anything you could complain about has an appropriate herb or combination of herbs that could be added to your bath.

Please do note that all herbs listed below should be dried, not fresh. Some fresh herbs (nettles for one) can be extremely irritating to the skin.

Herbs for Stiff Muscles and Aching Joints

A combination of sage and strawberry leaves, or sage and mugwort can be quite soothing in the case of stiff muscles and aching joints. Also try a combination of agrimony, chamomile, and mugwort (equal parts). Sassafras and burdock are also good for relaxing stiff achy muscles and joints. Or you may try this combination.

1 ounce sage (will stimulate the skin)

1 ounce mugwort (will ease sore muscles)

2 ounces chamomile (mild diaphoretic, makes you sweat)

1 ounce agrimony (eases sore muscles)

Mix all the herbs together thoroughly. Add 1 quart water and simmer for about 15-20 minutes. Strain out the herbs and pour the liquid into your bath.

Herbs for a Tonic Bath

Feeling a little off lately? Just can't seem to get going? A tonic bath might be just the ticket. A tonic is a substance that jump-starts the system to improve the health and tone up the body. This type of bath yields the most benefit if repeated each evening for several evenings in a row. Some herbs that have a tonic effect are: blackberry leaves, comfrey leaf and root, ginseng root, jasmine flowers, lavender, nettle leaf, orange, parsley, patchouli, raspberry leaf, rose petals, and strawberry leaf.

Try a mixing three parts jasmine flowers to one part orange blossoms, add water to cover, simmer 15 minutes, strain, and use the liquid in your bath. Another good tonic combo is equal parts of comfrey, alfalfa, parsley, and orange peel. After several evening soaks you just might end the day with a little energy surplus, and feel better overall.

Herbs to Relieve Tension

We have so much stress and tension in our modern world. Researchers have found that stress and tension can manifest themselves in all kinds of sickness and disease. Try a combination of your choice of any of the following to soothe the mind and body: catnip, chamomile, comfrey, hyssop, jasmine flowers, lemon balm, lavender flowers, linden flower, passion flower blossoms, roses, slippery elm bark, valerian roots, and violets. You can use equal parts of the herbs, or vary the proportions to suit your own needs.

½ ounce valerian root (sedative)

1 ounce catnip (calming)

1 ounce chamomile (calming)

1 ounce linden (sedative)

4-5 drops lavender essential oil

Simmer the valerian first—it's a root and need a bit more time. After about 10 minutes, add the rest of the herbs and simmer for another 10 minutes. Strain it all out and add the liquid to the bath, then add the lavender oil. This just may reduce you to a little puddle!

Herbs for a Stimulating Bath

Oh boy! You've had the day from—well, it's been some day! And you've still got several items on your to-do list—a PTA meeting to attend, and homework to help the kids with. A good idea now would be to take about 45 minutes for a bath. It'll be worth the time spent after all is said and done. A combination of any of these herbs can provide a wonderful lift at the end of a hectic day: basil, bay leaves, fennel, marjoram, rosemary, sage, savory, thyme, mint, nettle, peppermint, pine needles, lavender, lemon verbena, calendula, and vetivert root. Or you may try this particularly soothing combination:

2 parts peppermint

1 part rosemary

1 part nettle

½ part bay leaves

All of these herbs are stimulating and will give you a real boost in the bath. To start, mix them together, put generous handfuls of the herbs into a muslin bag, or into a wash cloth or several pieces of cheesecloth. Cover with water, and simmer for 10 minutes. Pour the liquid into the bath water, and use the herbs-in-a-bag to scrub down your body. You'll might just feel energized enough to take on the world again!

Herbs for Achy Feet

Almost all of us have had tired, achy feet at least once in our lives. When your feet hurt, it seems that everything hurts and nothing is working right. Here are some herbs that make a marvelous footbath. To take advantage of them, soak for 30 minutes or so, then talk someone into a foot massage. Try agrimony, burdock, lavender flowers, mustard seeds, sage, witch hazel, and wormwood to stimulate your feet and bring yourself back to a state of sanity.

To Soften and Cleanse

1 pound barley

4 pounds bran

8 ounces borage

This is an old recipe that I recipe rediscovered; however, you will need a large container to hold all of the bran. To start, combine all the ingredients and boil them in a large amount of water until everything is soft and mushy. Strain. Use the liquid in the bath, and the recovered barley mixture to scrub with. This is a great combination that will make your skin feel like silk.

Bath to Soften, Cleanse, and Soothe the Skin

Anise (cleansing)

Comfrey (soothing and softening)

Red clover (soothing)

Elder (softening)

Melilot (cleansing)

Mix equal parts of the herbs. (One ounce of each will make several baths.) Put two handfuls of the mixture into a large muslin bag, and simmer for 20 minutes. As always, the liquid goes into the bath and the herbs can be used to scrub with.

Hot Summer Nights Bath

You know the feeling—those unbearable summer nights when there's no breath of air, the humidity is up and you're sticking to your clothing, the sheets, and to yourself. Who can sleep when the nights are so miserable? Tempers are short and the night is interminably long. This mix will cool the body and the temper, and keep you feeling cool and refreshed—so maybe you can get some sleep after all.

Peppermint (cooling)

Rosemary (astringent)

Pennyroyal (astringent)

Houseleek (cooling)

This combo can be made by adding the herbs in equal parts. Cover them with water and simmer 10 minutes. On a hot summer night, a cool bath or shower would be just the ticket. In the shower, the liquid can be used as a rinse. The astringent herbs get rid of that "sticky" feeling that usually goes along with the dog days of summer, and the cooling herbs help the skin stay comfortable and refreshed.

A Soak for Oily Skin

Many of us suffer from overly oily skin. For those who have oily skin over most of their body, a nice bath with herbs that can cut the oil and act as an astringent is most helpful. Mix equal parts cornmeal, white willow bark, lemon grass, peppermint and witch hazel. Tie up a large handful in cheesecloth, a washcloth or muslin bag, add cold water to cover, bring to a boil, and simmer for ten minutes. First bathe or shower with soap to clean the skin and rinse. Then draw a fresh warm bath. Add the herb water to the bath. Soak for at least 20 minutes. Use the herb bag to thoroughly scrub the skin.

Dry or Chapped Skin Bath

1 part ginseng

1 part comfrey root

1 part marshmallow root

1 part almond meal

1 part oatmeal

Simmer the ginseng, marshmallow root and comfrey root first. After about 10 minutes add the rest and simmer an additional 10 minutes. Strain. The strained herbs can be used as a body scrub, and the liquid should be used in the bath.

Warm Soaking Bath for Colds or Flu

You're getting sick, you just know it. Your joints ache, your muscles hurt, your skin hurts, even your hair hurts! And you can never seem to get warm, even after piling on all the blankets in the house. A warm bath, using the following herbs, might be just what you need. The following herbs should help warm the body, ease achy muscles, and break up congestion.

1 ounce borage

2 ounces elder

1 ounce burdock

1 ounce mugwort

1/2 ounce bay leaves

1 ounce eucalyptus

1 ounce horehound

Mix the above herbs thoroughly. Cover 1 cup of the mixed herbs with water and simmer 10 minutes. Strain and add to your bath. The bath should be warm, not hot; the bathroom should also be warm, and you should have a comfy bathrobe to wrap up in when you're all done. You don't want to get chilled and ruin all the good you've just done.

Sensuous Bath

This is one to share with that special someone! Light candles, play some favorite erotic music, arrange flowers around, turn out the electric lights, and enjoy!

Rose petals

Lavender

Jasmine

Sandalwood

Chamomile

Mix a big handful of each of the herbs, and simmer the herbs in a couple of quarts of water—the exact amount depends on how many herbs you use; the herbs should be well-covered—for 15 minutes. Add 3-5 drops of the following essential oils to the liquid: ylang-ylang, sandalwood, clary sage, and lavender.

Deep Woods Refresher

Ever notice how invigorating and refreshing a forest smells? You can get the same thing in your bath. Just close your eyes and you won't have any trouble imagining yourself in a bubbling little brook, filled with the wonderful earthy fragrances of wood, earth, rocks, and plants of all kinds.

Last time I went walking in the woods, I started gathering bits and pieces of juniper, firs, conifers, and other evergreens. A few oak leaves also went into the mix. Later I used these to make a lovely scented bath, which immediately brought back the wonderfully intoxicating fragrance of the deep woods.

Next time you tramp through the woods, hike up the mountains or just wander through a meadow, watch for pine, juniper, cedar, or other evergreens. Gather some bark and leaves from the ground around these trees, and then when you need an instant refresher, get out your collection and add some sagebrush (which has the added benefit of being a natural deodorizer), meadowsweet, and some sweet woodruff. Then simmer in water—enough to cover. Strain the liquid into the tub and add a couple drops of cedar or pine essential oil. Sink down into the water, breathe deep, ahhh!

Eye-Opener Bath

No no! It can't be time to wake up already. It seems like you just laid down to sleep. But in fact it is time to start the day, and, groggily, you get up, bump you way into the kitchen, and spill water all over trying to make some coffee!

Here is a nice mix to help get those baby-blues open naturally, and to get that groggy mind functioning on a fuzzy winter morning.

Nettle

Savory

Lavender

Rosemary

Few drops of peppermint essential oil

Use equal parts of the herbs, cover with water, and simmer for the normal 10-20 minutes. Strain and pour liquid into the tub (use the herbs to scrub with if you're taking a shower, and rinse with the liquid). Add a drop or two (no more!) of peppermint oil to the bath, or to the herb bag.

Sleep-tight Bath

Oh those terrible nights when you toss and turn, and no matter what you do you just can't get to sleep. The mind is busy, and the muscles won't relax. Maybe it's worth the effort to get up and get a pleasant, warm, tranquil bath. You could just soak in the tub, or you could add some herbs that are almost guaranteed to get you to sleep.

Chamomile (relax muscles)

Linden (mild sedative)

Lemon verbena (eases insomnia)

Few drops of lavender essential oil

Mix the herbs together, and brew as usual (a handful of herbs, water to cover, simmer 10 minutes, strain). Make sure the water is comfortably warm in your bath, and add the herb liquid and lavender oil to the bath. Have the bathroom warm, as you don't want to get sleepily out of the tub and be jolted away by arctic-type temperatures. As you soak 15 or 20 minutes, sip a cup of chamomile tea. When you get into bed, sleep should not be quite so elusive. I've known people who have tried this and have barely been able to keep awake long enough to make it to the bed!

Final Herbal Bath Remedies

Aside from making health-giving teas, this concludes my brief sampling of what you can do with herbs.

In general, you can use almost any herbs in your bath. For example, lovely fragrances can be obtained with angelica root, bay leaves, cloves, jasmine and lavender flowers, lovage root, mint, orange leaves, flowers and peel, patchouli, pennyroyal, rose petals, rosemary, or sandalwood.

Sunburned skin can be soothed with aloe, comfrey, lettuce or witch hazel. Avocado, sorrel, tansy and elder should be considered if your skin is chapped or irritated. To improve skin tone try bay, chamomile, celery, salt, or vetivert.

Birch bark, comfrey root, germander, pansy, sassafras, thyme, or white willow bark may ease the "heartbreak of psoriasis." For puffiness try burdock, lavender, fennel, or chamomile. Almond meal, comfrey, oatmeal, and peppermint can help clear up pimples or mild acne.

Ambergris, comfrey, ginseng, gotu kola, jasmine, orange, patchouli, and rosemary are rejuvenating, while burdock, mugwort, pennyroyal, sage, and sassafras are relaxing.

In the end, be as creative as you dare. Try always to come up with your own favorite combinations. You'll find that an herbal bath, instead of a luxury, may well become a necessity.

Herbal Beauty Treatments

≈ By Caroline Moss ≈

D o you find yourself with so many commitments on the weekends that you can scarcely breathe? In today's hectic pace, we can often over-commit ourselves and find it difficult to relax. Whatever your circumstances I would urge you to try the following ideas for finding a simple, inexpensive way to relax and enjoy life.

Now, before I go on. You may find this article geared predominantly to women. However, I can assure you guys that it is just as relevant for you. Women do not have the monopoly on pampering: face packs and the like do wonders for male skin too. But if you feel that is not for you just leave out what you don't fancy and try the rest.

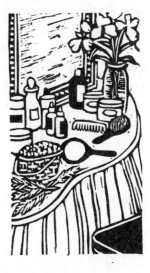

To get down to business, what we are going to do here is to have a luxurious 'health and beauty spa' session in the convenience of our own home, and at a fraction of the price of a 'real' health spa. In all the foods and treatments taken, full use will be made of herbs. No prepared cosmetics or foods need to be purchased.

To begin with, there are three focus areas we shall concentrate on: the external body (hair and skin), the internal body (food and drink), and the mind. In this program, a rough timetable for making progress will be suggested. You can, of course, pick out the bits that you want to follow and in an order which suits your own schedule.

On Rising

Try to sip a glass or two of cool mineral water as you get ready to greet the day. If you prefer a herb tea that is fine too. You should really try to avoid tea, coffee, and carbonated soft drinks, as well as, of course, as alcohol and cigarettes, if this day is to be a real treat for your body.

Now would also be the ideal time for a little exercise. Best would be to go out into the open air if possible, and jog or briskly walk. Do not, of course, get too enthusiastic about jogging if you are very overweight and have done little or no exercise recently. A brisk walk is almost as beneficial and a far wiser introduction to physical activity. Take things easy at first. Aim to exercise for around 15 minutes at a brisk pace. And finish your exercise session with a few minutes rest, sipping a glass of water.

If you have dry or normal hair, use this opportunity to massage in a little almond or coconut oil and leave on for twenty minutes or so. While the oil is working, have a warm, deep bath with a little added lavender oil to aid relaxation. Also add a pint of milk, which is a marvellous skin softener. So many of us shower nowadays for both speed and ecological reasons, but a deep bath is a real luxury in terms of relaxation and its beneficial effects on the skin.

If you have used an oil massage you will also need to wash your hair. Wash it with an herbal rinse to really freshen it up. Simply pour a pint of boiling water onto a handful of, preferably, fresh herbs and leave to steep for ten minutes. Strain, cool and use as final rinse. Rosemary or sage is best for dark hair, and chamomile is best to brighten fair hair. Such a rinse won't of course, have the immediate effect of commercial preparations but if you have blonde hair and use a chamomile rinse regularly it will really brighten it up in time.

While in the shower, finish off with a salt rub. Just take a handful of coarse sea salt and a teaspoonful of dried lavender and rub your skin briskly—arms, legs, body and (unless you have very sensitive skin) your face. Rinse well in the shower. Do not, of course, let the salt near any open cuts or your relaxed mood will end rather smartly. This is a beautifully invigorating activity and you will feel even better when you consider the price of abrasive skin rubs at the cosmetic counter!

If you prefer something a bit more gentle, just use coarse oatmeal mixed with a little milk as another good exfoliator. Also, before you dress, massage your skin with something soothing. For really cracked skin and hard areas on feet you could try a little almond oil. Or for your feet you could add two drops (no more) of tea tree oil to a teaspoonful of almond oil which will help heal any cracks and also inhibit athlete's foot. For very dry legs or arms you could add a couple of drops of your favourite scented oil, such as lavender. On less dry areas just use your own favorite body lotion.

If you have particularly dry or sore hands then a great restorative is to massage them with a combination of ground almonds (almond meal) and egg yolk. Afterwards, put on some cotton gloves if you have any, and leave the mixture in place for as long as you can— up to a couple of hours if possible. Then, wash you hands with warm water and finish off with a gentle hand cream. A little glycerine would be beneficial if your hands are particularly dry.

Breakfast

We want the Herbal Health Farm to rejuvenate the body as well as the soul and, therefore we will be eating enough to ensure we are happy and satisfied, but not so full as to overburden the digestive system.

For breakfast we need not be too prescriptive, but we might want to limit dairy products and eggs and rely on fruit, juice, and whole grains. Grains, of course, give the option of a wide variety of foods from breads and pancakes to oatmeal. Oats in particular are a marvellous grain to incorporate into the diet, as they are beneficial to the heart and can help the body control cholesterol. If you choose some form of grains, do be moderate in your use of sweetener.

Another good breakfast option would be a smoothie—a nutritious and delicious drink which makes a complete breakfast in itself. Try whizzing in your blender a banana, a few strawberries, two tablespoonsful of plain yoghurt, and enough orange juice to make a drinking consistency. The banana, orange juice, and yoghurt makes a good, basic base to which you can add your own choice of fruit. The flavor can be perked up by the addition of a few sprigs of lemon balm, mint, or hyssop leaves, and a bigger nutritional hit can be made by adding an egg and any vitamins or supplements (such as wheatgerm or lecithin) which your doctor or health adviser has recommended. Smoothies, particularly thos with ripe bananas, do not normally need any sweetening; but if your taste goes in that direction, or if you have added some particularly tart berries, then by all means add a little honey. Do note that raw eggs should not be taken by young children, the elderly, pregnant women, or anyone concerned about the slight risks involved.

Morning

So you are washed and breakfasted—what is next? Since you have benefitted your complexion by getting the oxygen pumping during your exercise, and since you have washed and exfoliated your face while bathing and showering, you can now, unless you are over 50 or with very sensitive skin, deep clean your face. The reason I exclude the more mature or sensitive skin is that a facial steam is, while beneficial to others, too aggressive for such faces and would cause more harm than good in terms of broken veins and the like. For others, however, it is useful to put a handful of herbs (fresh or dried) in a large bowl, pour on boiling water, and lean over the bowl with a towel over your head for about five minutes or so.

For this deep steam-cleansing, try using, alone or in combination: chamomile, comfrey, rose, lavender, or lemon verbena . These herbs will give the skin a beautiful scent and will stimulate blood vessels close to the skin's surface. Afterwards, rinse your face with lukewarm water—never icy as is sometimes recommended, as this can damage the skin—and dab any open pores or blemishes with witch-hazel.

You might then like to try a face mask. As a highly beneficial remedy for your skin as well as your psyche, some great preparations can be made from fresh, natural ingredients depending on skin type. You can find more complicated preparations than these but I aim for simplicity.

To begin, before applying any mask, rinse your face with very warm, but not scalding, water. Massage the preparation on gently, avoiding the eye area. Relax for fifteen minutes with a cool, used teabag, or a slice of potato or cucumber over each eye and your feet raised slightly above your head (just use a couple of pillows under your ankles). Really pamper yourself with some lovely music and a scented candle. After quarter of an hour or so, rinse off the mask with plenty of warm water.

For very dry skin—combine a teaspoonful each of almond oil, honey, oats, and egg yolk.

For moderately dry skin—combine a teaspoonful each of honey, oats and egg yolk, and a little mashed banana.

For normal skin—combine a little lightly beaten egg white with a sprinkling of oats and a little mashed banana.

For oily skin—mash a little papaya (an excellent astringent) and combine with natural yoghurt and a few drops of lemon juice.

After rinsing, dry gently and wipe over face and neck with a herbal infusion made in the same way as the hair rinse—that is, by pouring a couple of cups of boiling water onto a handful of herbs, leaving to infuse for ten minutes, straining and cooling. Use lavender for a dry or normal skin, rose petals alone or with rosemary for normal skin, and mint with a dash of lemon juice for oily skin.

For the rest of the morning do something to maintain and enhance your mood. That is, take the telephone off the hook and read, take a stroll, rest, play or listen to music or simply potter about the house. A word of warning, however; although the television may seem to be relaxing, you will feel much more rested if you don't watch, so try giving it a break for a day.

Lunch

After your selfish morning, for lunch, as with breakfast, you need to concentrate on grains, fruits, and vegetables. Maybe you should try a large salad with sprigs of herbs such as fennel, chives, parsley, or mint added to your usual greens for extra flavor and nutritional value. In cooler weather a fresh vegetable soup is a comforting option. Again, the addition of fresh, finely chopped herbs stirred in at the last minute or sprinkled on top make a very plain dish far more flavorful and appealing.

Afternoon

The idea is to have a complete break and it is certainly no crime to simply rest on your bed or read a book. However, if you wish to use this free time to have some lasting health and beauty benefits then why not have a 'herby' afternoon with one of the following suggested activities:

Design or modify a herb garden—prepare for this activity by reading plenty of inspirational and instructive library books, herb nursery catalogues, and a notebook and graph paper for lists and sketch plans

Revisit your recipe books or try new ones and list lots of unfamiliar recipes to try making the best use of fresh herbs

Gain inspiration and insights by looking at the lives of some prominent herbalists such as early Europeans John Gerard and Nicholas Culpeper or 20th century writers, practitioners, and growers.

Make a large batch of potpourri—you will feel wonderfully productive at the end when you have a generous pile of bags, tied with smart ribbons or country twine, ready for your own home or to give away

Clearly some of these projects require some forward thinking to ensure you have books and materials at hand but all, I am sure you will agree, would be a delightful way of passing a few restful, uninterrupted hours.

Throughout this time, whenever you feel hugner, try to stick to water or herb teas and crudites (pieces of raw vegetable such as carrot or celery sticks) or fruit. Avoid all junk food whenever you feel the urge.

Evening

For supper try a large mixed fruit salad. Just use whatever fruits you wish. You could have a traditional cut up fruit salad to serve with a spoon in its own juice. However, I prefer just to have the pieces of fruit in their natural state. You might like to serve a couple of tablespoons of Greek (strained plain) yoghurt flavoured with a dab of honey and a few very finely chopped leaves of lemon balm. A couple of oat cookies would make this rather more filling.

After a leisurely evening try to be in bed by 10 o'clock at the latest with nothing stronger than a milky drink if you like such beverages. Milk is recommended as a bed-time drink as it can induce drowsiness by directing blood from the brain to the stomach. If you don't care for milk then either chamomile or lemon verbena tea are mild sedatives.

I hope that if you follow even some of the ideas you will enjoy a beautiful, self-centered day using plenty of herbs for skin care and sustenance.

Herb
Crafts

Casting the Circle

∾ By K.D. Spitzer ∾

Spirit Smoke Smudging and Censing

Burning herbs, resins, roots, grasses and tree needles is an ancient and important part of sacred ritual. It calls for the power of the plant and the element of air to create sacred space in ceremony. The sacred fire and the salamanders that live within lend energy to this process. Smoke is a powerful purification; and a column of smoke sends our prayers out into the universe and returns the answers back to us. Sylphs and angels dance in the air around us when we call on them and their element to clear energy in our ritual space and around our ritual tools. They lend their spirit to the spellworking of magic.

Air is the element of the intellect. If you have had difficulty in the past getting a smudge stick to light, it is

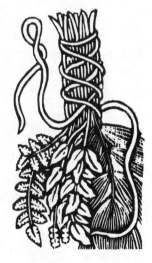

most likely that you have not been intellectually focused on your task. You need to take a deep breath, center your thinking and then try again. It may also be that it was not well-made to begin with, or perhaps, the universe is indicating that it is time for you to prepare your own.

Sacred smoke has a traditional place in cultures around the world and is used not only to clear sacred space for ritual or offerings to the gods and goddesses, but also to heal the body, lighten a heavy spirit, or focus the mind. Utilizing the antiseptic properties of particular plants, healers burn them in the sickroom to dispel germs and evil humours in the air, or in public places to repel disease brought in by the unwashed and the poor.

It is common in some parts of the world to stand and bathe in frankincense smoke for daily hygiene, or to reduce the joint pain of rheumatism, or to increase circulation. Myrrh and other resins are burned to relax the body and fight insomnia.

The ancient Egyptians were fond of fragrant smoke and used it to scent the air and create a sense of well-being. There is much archeological evidence that even three centuries b.c., the Egyptians used scented smoke to perfume and enhance their environment. They used fragrances to increase their aesthetic appreciation, their sensuality, and their joy in living. And they hadn't even heard of aromatherapy!

With a little time and trouble, it is easy enough for you to create your own fragrant world. Consider the tradition you are following or creating, and think about the ancient rituals of your own ancestors. Experiment with different scents and begin to understand the power of plants grown in nearby woods or your own garden.

Prepared smudge sticks are readily available in new age shops, book stores, health food stores, and herb shops. It is sold as "sage" and is often mixed with cedar and sweetgrass—though it is not sage at all, but prairie sage or sage brush. These wands are fairly pricey and unless you are following some sort of American Indian tradition or live in the west, there is no reason why you should use them for smudging. The natural habitat for most of the Native American smudging herbs popularly used today is the desert, the prairie, and the west coast.

Making Your Own Smudge-Stick

If you live elsewhere, it is far more potent to gather your own local and native plants to use in your ceremonies. These plants already resonate with the same local vibrations as yourself and will readily lend themselves in harmony to your rituals. It is a simple matter to harvest or wildcraft the small amounts that you need, tie them tightly in a bundle with soft cotton yarn, and hang them to dry. As they dry, they will shrink and loosen in the bundle which makes for better burning.

In general, however, it is important to follow these simple rules in wildcrafting.

1. Always be certain of your plant's identity.

2. If wildcrafting for any reason, be sure there are sister plants in the same area and only harvest up to 20%.

3. Never strip the plant, but only take a small amount from the tips so the plant will continue to grow. Some choose to harvest only a leaf from each plant. Never harvest from the largest or the smallest plants.

4. If you can use your finger tips to pinch off what you need, you will be in better communion with the plant. Metal often leaves a residue that turns color on the cut ends.

5. Be sure to ask permission of the plant beforehand and leave a small offering to the gnomes to say thanks. A shiny penny, a pretty rock, a flower, or some grain will do.

Lay several small botanicals—from 4" to 6" in length—together, lining up the stem ends. You can leave the berries on the juniper branches, and tuck a piece of lavender, sage, or rosemary in the middle. Tie the stems with a piece of cotton string, winding it in a spiral around the bundle of herbs. Make sure you tuck in the ends so they are not exposed. Then wind back down towards the stems, crisscrossing what you previously wound. Tie securely and hang upside down to dry. This will take several weeks, so allow enough time before using.

By making your own smudging wands, you can tie together herbs that have special meaning for each ceremony that you perform. Use herbs that have special meaning for each Sabbat, Esbat, or goddess you are invoking. Consider using plants from your herb garden; sprigs of lavender, rosemary or garden sage make special additions to your bundle. It is important to start your own traditions based on the work you are doing and not blindly follow another's. There is more power in any tool you bring to a ritual if you have created it yourself. This is also true for medicines and foods.

Useful Plants for Smudging

Some of the following plants are native to US soil and have a western tradition in Native American ceremony. Others are indigenous to the East coast and have a healing tradition going back before colonial times. Many plants were brought by European immigrants. All have a traditional use in smudging. For some, their use can be traced back to ancient times.

Conifers

Conifers are trees often used in smudging. California incense cedar (Calocedrus descurrens) is generally preferred by those living in the west. In the northeast, northern white cedar is a good choice and can probably be found in your front or side yard as a wind break. Thuja occidentalis is also known as eastern white cedar. The word Thuja has its roots in the Greek words for "to fumigate" and also "to sacrifice." Fragrant, resinous woods were commonly used as the fuel in altar sacrifices so that the offering drifted to the gods and goddesses on an aromatic smoke. It also served to cover the scent of animal sacrifices. The Egyptians favored cedar aromatics, believing they had magical powers which could be revealed by special incantations. They even burned it after lovemaking to restore mental harmony.

A useful tree, eastern white cedar is very rich in vitamin C and teas have been prepared using foliage and bark. Legend says it probably saved Jacques Cartier and his crew from scurvy. Distilled cedar oil is poisonous to ingest, but an excellent vermifuge. Its green branches are often placed on hot rocks in saunas or sweat lodges. They have even been bound together to make an fragrant besom. Use any of the cedars to clear and consecrate your magic wand.

Eastern red cedar (Juniperus virginiana) is quite widespread on the East coast. This aromatic wood has been used commercially in fence posts and pencils. Its berries are eaten by many kinds of wildlife, including the cedar waxwing which takes it name from these berries. If you can't find one in the wild, look in the pet department for bags of red cedar shavings which smolder quite nicely on charcoal.

Also very aromatic is the dwarf, or common, juniper (Juniperus communis). This low-growing and prickly shrub is found cultivated as foundation plantings or growing wild as scrub in meadows and fields or along timber lines. Its berries when ripe are used to flavor soups and stews, and especially as a seasoning for wild game. They also lend a distinctive aroma and tang to gin. In the field, the berries are prized by game birds like grouse and pheasant, as well as other wildlife. The dried berries and wood are both suitable for smudging. Juniper was especially prized for inducing trance, by not only the ancient Greeks and Romans, but also the shamans among the Germanic tribes and the tribes along the foothills of the Himalayas.

The cedars and junipers clear negativity and call the attention of the goddess and bod. Their scent is sweet and calming, and they have an ancient tradition in Old World temples. However, the cedars can cause allergic reaction, so be sure of the effect on you before using it for ceremony.

Pine

Pine burned as a smudge is very cleansing, vigorous and purifying. It is sacred to the Celtic god, Cernunnos. It carries intention in its smoke and brings peacefulness. Pine needles and bark are loaded with vitamin C, and were brewed as tea for colds. And even the seeds are edible.

Eastern white, or Weymouth, pine (Pinus strobus) used to be the most valuable tree in the Northeast, used for masts and lumber. Red pine (Pinus resinosa) is also found all over New England. Pinon Pine (Pinus edulis) is most popular for smudging in the west. Pitch pine (Pinus rigida) is an excellent source for pine resin, which should be harvested when the pitch is dry. Pine resin can be used alone for smudging, and ground and blended with other herbs it makes a good altar incense. Pine needles make a resinous and aromatic smudge but they are often combined with other conifers and herbs in a bundle. Try using with lavender sprigs or garden sage.

Other local conifers also are suitable for smudging. Any variety of pine and fir can be used; the spruces and hemlock, larch and tamarack all lend their needles and resin for sacred smoke. Resin can be harvested from any of the conifers; be sure to take only the beads that are dry and do not damage the tree. The advantage of all these trees is that they are green the year round and thus readily available. In many ways they are the guardians of the earth's energies.

Herbals

Bay laurel (Laurel nobilis) was used as an ancient incense in Greek and Roman temples dedicated to Apollo. The High Priestess at Delphi burned bay and juniper, along with henbane, to enhance powers of divination. Not only do the leaves represent greatness and glory, but the tree is a traditional symbol for personal protection. Thunder and lightning cannot withstand its powerful plant energy. Its smoke will carry requests to the goddess. It is not hardy in the north, but can be wintered over easily in a tub. It may grow slowly the first couple years but then will take off if well cared for.

Wild California bay (Umbellaria californica) has a medicinal tradition with west coast Indians as a smoke inhalant for colds and flu. It is also suitable for magick and will lend its powers to prosperity spells as well. Prairie sage (Artemesia tridentata) has a wonderfully clean, sharp scent which is calming, and helps with focusing. It grows in poor soil and in an arid climate. It is best harvested in the spring before flowering. This is the main plant in the sage bundles sold most everywhere and is probably your first experience with sacred smoke. It clears negativity and guards sacred space. It is often called desert mugwort.

White sage (Salvia apiana) is related to garden sage, and its white leaves are generally burned alone or loosely on charcoal, rather than bound together. It has a sharp scent that is soothing and it is very good for clearing ceremonial objects. It has been grown successfully in northern climates, although it is native to hot, dry climates.

Sweetgrass (Hierochloe odorata) can be grown in your own garden and I recommend it. Found in Europe as well as North America, it is part of both cultural traditions. Symbolic of the hair of the goddess, or the grandmother, sweetgrass is usually sold in braids and will keep its scent for years if properly stored. It used to be woven into small baskets, and quite often these lidded baskets still retain their fragrance long after they were made. Occasionally an old handkerchief basket can be found in antique markets. Cloth hankies can still be scented by storage in these baskets.

Sweetgrass's light sweet scent attracts positive energy. It can be burned for a blessing and to offer up a prayer. It is very soothing and grounding. Make room in your herb cupboard for this herb, and use it often.

Sweet Fern (Comptonia peregrina) is not really a fern at all, but a small shrub. It grows in dry, sunny locations and is easily found on a walk in the woods or meadow. Its unique scent is released by the heat of the Sun and will touch off memories of long, lazy summer days. Sweetly scented, it has been used as a strewing herb, as well as a vermifuge and aromatic (along with lavender) in the linen closet. Sweet Fern brings with it a grounding energy that is light and soothing, but warm in feeling. It will help with focusing. Bundle or burn it loose on a charcoal tablet.

Herbs from your garden have a special place in smudge sticks, ground and blended into incense, or burned alone. Many common herbs that are notable today for culinary uses have ancient symbolism in magic or as intercessors to the goddess. Grow any of the following for ready accessibility in smudging.

Basil (Ocymum basilium) is a very versatile herb and when smudged can be used to cleanse negativity. It helps to prepare you for something new, so it is useful for self-initiation. Also smudge with basil for courage.

Hyssop (Hyssopus officinalis) is a strong herb for cleansing and protection from negative energies. Add a single sprig to your smudge stick. Make an infusion and use in the rinse water when washing ritual robes. Bind several springs with leather and use to clear your sacred space either by burning or using as a wand for spurging. Burning hyssop is a powerful enhancer while practicing reiki.

Garden sage (Salvia officinalis) is excellent for personal purification. Smudge yourself with sage to cleanse your spirit and prepare for ritual work. Like basil and mugwort, it is very versatile and very important, with varied uses in cooking, medicine, ceremony and magic.

Lavender (Lavendula officinalis) brings a sense of mysticism to ceremony. Tuck a sprig into any smudge stick. At the Summer Solstice, be sure to use several sprigs (along with St John's Wort) to cleanse the ritual space. Burn it by itself to bring calmness and peace of mind. It's especially suitable for special meditations. Use it as a wand for spurging sacred circles. In some cultures, it was burned in the birthing room as an antiseptic, a calmative for the mother, and a welcoming blessing for the babe.

Rosemary (Rosmarinus officinalis) mixed with Juniper will purify the air where it is burned. It is a protection against evil and frightening dreams. It's a good herb to clean your aura. As the herb of remembrance, it was burned as incense at funerals. It enhances the "sacred" at every ritual. Tie with ribbons and gold to enhance and honor its powers. This herb is a special occult herb, and it combines well with others.

Thyme (Thymus vulgaris) is another special herb of protection. Its smoke will clear the air of old energies and is perfect for smudging a new home and to bring the family together. Thyme can call the fairies and was once used as a funeral herb. Its Latin name Thuja suggests its use on ancient altars.

Mugwort (Artemesia vulgaris) has an ancient reputation as an herb to smudge when scrying; it aids in visualization and in developing a trance. It can also protect you at that time. Mugwort was so important that it was the first herb mentioned in the Lacnunga, a surviving scrap of an herbal from early Anglo Saxon times. Its powers are many. Burn it at the Summer Solstice and other times to help in letting go. It's important to woman as it can mark transition and bring balance in key life changes. It can help relax the body into sleep and activate the body to begin healing.

Elecampane (Inula helenium) is another respected Celtic herb that is easily cultivated in the garden. The root is the important part of the plant and has a strong healing tradition. However, it also has a long tradition as an incense. The plant represents the Sun and is used as part of a Summer Solstice incense. It is best used in the winter when the days are short, helping with the winter blues and cabin fever. It restores balance and harmony in the gloomy days when the sun is struggling to return its position of dominance.

Coriander (Coriandrum sativum) adds a wonderful spicy scent to incense mixtures. Although grown and valued around the world, it grows easily in the cold northeast as its seeds have time to develop during the short season. Coriander aids in calming tension and reducing chronic headache pain. Its fragrant seeds restore harmony where there has been anger, and its pleasing scent creates a comfortable atmosphere.

There are, of course, other herbs that grow in North American gardens that have a tradition of incense burning. The best of incense mixtures have at least fifty percent of their bulk in resins. Usually these are frankincense, myrrh, and copal. It takes some time and energy to gather enough resin from local conifers to sustain this proportion. Propolis is a natural waxy resin produced by bees and you may be able to purchase it from a local beekeeper. Otherwise it can be purchased from a natural foods store.

Keep careful records in every experiment, otherwise you will never remember your recipes. Be sure and record when and where you harvested your herbs and any other pertinent data you will need to recall later. Label the jars you have stored your mixtures in. The herbs need to be dry before securing with a lid; otherwise they will mildew. Plan ahead. Mixtures need to sit for a week or so—even when the herbs are dry—so the scents have a chance to blend.

You don't need to use an entire charcoal tablet when you burn incense. You can use the sharp point of a knife to break the tablet into pieces. Put it on a cutting board first. Hold it with tweezers to light. You only need small amounts of incense at a time. There's no point in burning so much that you set off the smoke detectors or cause nose bleeds!

Use your incense to strengthen your spiritual energy, create sacred space, and provide a calm and harmonious environment. Explore its use in healing, relieving insomnia, and enhancing your dreams. Enjoy the pleasure of its scent.

Indigo Dyeing

≫ By K.D. Spitzer ≪

*I*n his Commentaries, one of the first remarks that Caesar makes about his conquest of Gaul and Britain was that the natives had painted themselves blue in order to frighten their enemies. The color blue was not unknown to the Romans—they imported indigo from India and Egypt for fabrics and inks—but it was relatively rare and costly. For the Britains (and other barbaric Celts) to have enough blue dye stuff to paint themselves was impressive enough, and of course, the fact that they were naked, except for their sandals, was an astonishingly fierce and terrorizing sight.

That we are still talking about it two-thousand years later is partly because these men were such ferocious fighters, but also because the search for dyes, the overwhelming need for color (along with the driving desire for

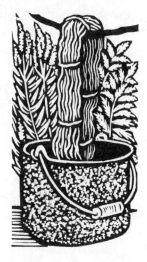

spices) has always been a means and excuse for private empire building among the ambitious and daring. Early Britains, for instance, had an established and thriving dye trade that enabled them to paint themselves blue in battle.

In fact, for all of recorded history, vicious wars were fought to secure various component parts of the dye industry—including alum and other mordants, indigo, and woad. In the Mediterranean, the Phoenicians committed economic suicide and eradicated a entire sea snail species (Murex) pandering to the egos of the rich and powerful because this tiny snail produced minute amounts of the color purple. The resulting dye was so expensive that it was affordable only to the most wealthy kings and emperors; purple is still considered the color of royalty. The coup de grace to this dying (and dyeing) industry in fact was administered by invading armies, and by the early Middle Ages the sea snails and Tyrian purple were gone. Certainly by the Renaissance, the urgent European need for color was outstripped only by the insatiable and rapacious need for money and the territory which it brought.

The History of Indigo

Indigo dyeing was an established and lucrative trade in India well before Caesar and his legions marched through the known world, probably dating back to 4000 b.c. according to Sanskrit records. Early Egyptians (2000 b.c.) understood the use of metallic salts to adhere color to fiber. Indeed the dye trade emerged hand in hand with woven textiles, and around the world, including China, evidence supports that it happened well before recorded history. Most cultures produced a vivid blue cloth of some sort.

Indigofera tinctoria, or indigo, is a perennial shrub originating in southeast Asia and growing to five feet in some climates. It can be grown as an annual, but in the cold Northeast, the season is not long enough for it to flower and thus develop dye pigment. When properly grown, the plant produces quite the pigment punch, so it might be surprising that it wasn't until the 17th century that it began to enjoy favor in Europe. The reason for this can be found with those ferocious Britains. They managed to successfully protect their thriving woad trade with the same fierceness they brought to their territorial wars.

Isatis tinctoria, or woad, was still used to make blue dye even after the introduction of indigo by the West Indies Company, a British company. It was possibly because European dyers did not understand the techniques of indigo dyeing or extraction of pigments in indigo dyeing, but early dyers' records show that the two blues were commonly combined. In fact, the pigment in both blues is indigotin, but indigo plants have a lot more of it than woad. Indigo is a perennial in warm climates and the annual woad can develop into a pernicious weed.

There are varieties of indigo found throughout the world, and certainly evidence exists that the color blue found a place even in the dye repertoire of the ancient Americas. The particular plant that produced this blue was Indigo suffruticosa (Guatemalan indigo), and today it can be successfully grown from seed in colder climates, producing enough dye to please the most avid weaver or dyer. Polygonum tinctorium (Japanese indigo) can also be grown for dye in colder zones and is the basis for a thriving dye industry in Japan. Indigo is woven into folk culture there with traditional health safeguards provided by the herb.

Purchasing seeds for either of these two plants from a reputable business is preferable to wild harvesting, because then you know you have the plants that produce pigment. You only need to purchase seeds once, as you can easily harvest the seeds from your own plants thereafter. False indigo or wild indigo (Baptisia australis) are wildly beautiful plants for the garden, but produce no indigotin, even when the seeds are as a dye plant. You must certainly take care in what you buy.

An Indigo Dye Bath

It is a little tricky to develop an indigo dye bath. This pigment is not water soluble, and it is not interested in bonding to fibers. The extracted pigment, after certain processes requiring ammonia (traditionally stale urine from a preadolescent male child) and wheat bran, becomes the dye bath called indigo white. Oxygen is required to turn the color to indigo blue, but the result is a rich and long-lasting hue that seems to be the result of magic.

You can purchase powdered indigo from weaving suppliers or you can grow your own plants, harvest the leaves (the part of the plant with the pigment), process them and finally dye your fibers. Powdered indigotin can be mixed with lard to produce a warrior's body paint. The Society for Creative Anachronism can provide designs that are appropriate to a fierce warrior. Whether you are using woad or indigo plants, the pigment you extract is the same. Indigo will just provide more of it with less.

Fresh Leaves Recipe

You can begin to harvest leaves from your indigo or woad plants when they begin to flower. There is maximum pigment at that time, and it's all in the leaves. It's good to have a waxing moon in a fixed sign for picking. Rita Buchanon suggests picking only one-third of the leaves on each plant so that you can continue your harvest for several weeks. Of course this will make the plants bushier, thus producing more leaves. You need to begin and end on the same day to be successful with this recipe.

If you harvest eight ounces of indigo, you'll need to quadruple that for woad. Chop the leaves coarsely and cover with hot water in a jar. The woad water can be almost boiling. Cover the jar and let stand for about an hour. Then put the whole jar into a hot water bath, double boiler style. Slowly bring the temperature of the dye bath up to 160° for about two hours. Be careful about this because raising the temperature too quickly will leave you with beautiful browns and golds, and not a blue in sight.

Strain off the liquid and squeeze the leaves. You can discard the leaves or use them in a new dye bath with mordanted wool for those lovely browns and golds.

For the blues, add a tablespoon of baking soda or a non-sudsy ammonia to make the solution alkaline. At this point you have the precursor to indigo, but now you need to add a little oxygen to the solution, so pour it back and forth between two jars for several minutes. Dissolve one tablespoons of Rit brand Color Remover—which is sodium hydrosulfite—in a jar of warm water. Blend it with the dye water and stir it well. Let it sit in a pan of warm water for a couple of hours. It should look yellow.

Make sure your yarns are we—they do not need mordant. Let them soak in the dye bath for 20 to 25 minutes. If you lift them into the air and then dip into the dye bath, you should be able to deepen the color. Repeat this several times until the yarn is whatever shade you desire. You can dye additional batches until the pigment is exhausted. This will only dye a small amount of yarn—about four ounces at most.

Powdered Indigo Recipe

Using a quart jar, mix one teaspoon of powder indigo with one teaspoon of Rit brand Color Remover in a pint of warm water. The indigo may be a solid brick which can be powdered with a hammer. Put in a plastic baggie, and leaving one end open for escaping air, pound it with a hammer to break it up. Do a good job as the unbroken pieces will not dissolve. Let the mixture sit for fifteen minutes or so. Then fill the jar with non-sudsy and unscented ammonia. At this point you can let the solution sit undisturbed over night or until the solution becomes clear and slightly yellow. This is the dye solution; there will be sediment in the bottom which is the undissolved indigo.

Fill your dye pot with hot water; this should be a non-reactive metal pot large enough to hold your yarns. Add one-half tea-spoon of the Rit brand Color Remover and let stand for fifteen minutes. This will eliminate the undissolved oxygen.

Carefully add the indigo solution without including the sed-iment. Add wet yarns, but do not agitate; make sure they are completely immersed. After ten to twenty minutes, you can remove the fibers and expose to the air. Repeat until you have the desired depth color. This will dye about four ounces of wool.

There is such a mystery to the process of dyeing with indigotin—whether your source is indigo or woad. One minute your yarns are white and you are despairing that you have wasted your efforts and then you pull them from the solution and before your eyes they begin to turn green and then blue.

The magic has worked again.

Suppliers for Dye Herbs

Sunnybrook Farms Nursery in Chesterland, Ohio. 216-729-7232

Well-Sweep Herb Farm in Port Murray, New Jersey. 210-852-5390

Suppliers for Natural Dye Stuffs in East Berlin, Pennsylvania.

Rumplestiltskin in Sacramento, California.

Earth Guild in Asheville, North Carolina. 800-327-8448

The Magic of Herb Sachets

✤ By Deborah C. Harding ✤

According to Webster's Unabridged Dictionary, a sachet is "a scent bag or perfume cushion to be laid among handkerchiefs, garments, etc., to perfume them." That is what everyone recognizes as a sachet. They are pretty little bags filled with herbs and flowers that lend their scent to clothing and linens, but sachets can also be highly magical objects.

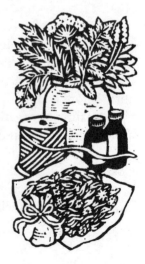

Sachets have been made and used by many cultures and in many ages. Romans used bath sachets; bags filled with herbs, oils, and other substances and prize for their scent and skin-softening traits. Sachets were also used during the Middle Ages. Cities during this time had no sanitary sewers, and city odors were, at times, very unpleasant. People would carry a scented handkerchief, a tussy mussy (a bouquet of dried or fresh flowers and herbs), and sachets that they would sniff when the stench became overpowering.

The American Indians make a type of sachet, but theirs are more religious in nature. Called ties, they contain shredded, dried tobacco, sage, cedar, or sweetgrass. The dried plants are placed in a small square of fabric that is usually red, representing honor, and tied with thread or cording. These sacred herbs of the Native Americans are set apart to be used in ceremonies and to be given to honored guests as gifts.

Scented Sachets

Making sachets is an easy process. You will need a small amount of loosely woven fabric (cotton is best), a piece of one-eighth inch wide ribbon, dried herbs, flowers, and scented oils.

To make a scented sachet cut a 4" x 4" square of fabric. Use calico or muslin for simplicity or you can use satin to make an eloquent sachet. Use pinking shears to notch the edges of the squares or use a fray guard (liquid applied to the edges of fabric to prevent fraying). Place the scented fill or potpourri (about one to two tablespoons) in the center of the fabric and pull up all the corners to create a bundle. Wrap a 12" strand of ribbon around the gathered edges so that the bundle is totally closed, and tie in a bow.

There are several options that can be undertaken to make the sachet more pleasing to the eye. Add dried or silk flowers by tying them under the ribbon or hot gluing them to the center of the bow. Hand stitch a strand of strung beads or ric-rac to the fabric before adding the potpourri. Instead of pinking the edges of your fabric, sew gathered lace trim on the wrong side of the fabric before filling and tying.

Another way of making a scented sachet is to take a large cookie cutter in any shape and trace the shape on the wrong side of the fabric. Cut out two and sew them together, wrong sides out, leaving a one-inch opening in the side or top. Turn your sachet right side out. Take a funnel and place it in the opening. Fill the sachet with potpourri and then, by hand, sew the opening shut.

Potpourri

Potpourri can be purchased in most craft stores, but you can also make your own. You will need dried herbs and flowers, essential oils, and a fixative. A fixative is a substance that holds the scent of the essential oils. Most fixatives can be purchased at craft stores. Oak moss, stag moss, and orris root are the most common fixatives. One can be substituted for the other in any of these recipes. Find which one is the cheapest and use it.

Here are a few scented potpourris that are easy to make:

Rose/Lavender Potpourri

3 tablespoons orris root

8 drops lavender oil

6 drops rose geranium oil

2 cups lavender blossoms

1 cup rose petals

Place the orris root in a plastic recloseable bag and drop in the oils. Shake to combine. Pour this mixture into a plastic bowl and add the blossoms and petals. Mix well.

Moth Potpourri

1 cup rosemary

1 cup vetiver, cut up

1 cup pennyroyal

10 whole bay leaves, crushed

1 cup crumbled cedar shavings

3 drops rosemary oil

4 drops pennyroyal oil

This potpourri is good for keeping moths and other insects away from clothing. In a bowl combine the rosemary, vertiver, pennyroyal, and bay leaves. In this case, the cedar shavings are the fixative. In a recloseable plastic bag combine the cedar shavings (roll with a rolling pin to crush well) and oil. Shake to mix well and add to ingredients in the bowl. Mix well.

Scented sachets are also good for producing a good night's sleep. These are more commonly called bed sachets. To make bed sachets you will need to produce two identical scented sachets and instead of tying them separately, cut the ribbon about 16" long and tie each sachet to each end of the ribbon. Hang the ribbon over the bedpost or on the headboard. A bed sachet can be made flat and be tucked inside the bed pillow. Make two eight by four-inch rectangles from fabric, sew them together leaving a one-inch gap in a side. Turn right side out, fill with potpourri, and stitch shut. To make this little pillow sachet appealing, sew gathered lace on two sides. Make sure the potpourri for a flat bed sachet doesn't stick out of the fabric to scratch the sleeper. Dried herbs can be very sharp and scratchy.

Here are a few potpourris to put in a sleep sachet. They will aid in sound sleep, dispel nightmares, and give magical dreams to the sleeper. The method of combining the potpourri is the same for both. In a recloseable plastic bag combine oak moss with essential oils. Close and shake well. In a plastic or glass bowl combine dried material and add oak moss and oils. Mix well.

Lavender Sweet Dream Potpourri

¼ cup oak moss

4 drops lavender oil

4 drops rose oil

1/2 cup chamomile flowers

¾ cup lavender buds

½ cup hops

¼ cup dried rose petals

Herbal Sweet Dream Potpourri

¼ cup oak moss

5 drops lemon balm oil

½ cup chamomile flowers

¼ cup catnip

¾ cup lemon balm leaves

½ cup hops

Make your own dream pillow blends by using one or more of the following herbs with oak moss and a corresponding essential oil.

Anise: Banishes nightmares

Chamomile: Induces restful sleep and sweet dreams

Hops: Induces sleep

Lavender: Induces sleep and prophetic dreams

Calendula: Induces sleep and prophetic dreams

Peppermint: Induces sleep and prophetic dreams

Rosemary: Banishes nightmares

Thyme: Banishes nightmares

Bath Sachets

Bath Sachets can also be called bath bags. These too are easy to make from a terricloth washcloth and ribbon. Take a terricloth wash rag and fold down one end about one-half inch, and sew right along the edge to make a casing for the ribbon to come through. This will be the top. Now fold in half and, starting under the casing (not including the casing), on one side, stitch down that side, along the bottom to the fold. Turn the bag right side out. Cut 1 yard of one-eighth inch ribbon and secure a safety pin through one end. Slide this through the casing so that it comes out on the other side. If you pull the ribbon on both ends the bath sachet should shut. Now place about two table-spoons of your bath potpourri into a coffee filter. Bring up the edges, twist into a bundle, and secure with a rubber band. Place this inside your terricloth bath sachet. Putting herbs directly into the terricloth sachet makes cleanup very difficult. This way, just take the insert out and throw it away. Hook the bag over the water spigot of your bathtub and run warm water. The bath sachet works as a "tea bag" to lend scent and softening qualities to the water.

Bath potpourri does not call for a fixative, since long-lasting scent is not required. The procedure for making the potpourri is the same for all. Combine the ingredients and place about one-quarter cup in each coffee filter.

Here are a few bath potpourris for you to use. These make great gifts for family and friends:

Itchy dry skin Potpourri

½ cup chamomile flowers

½ cup calendula petals

½ cup comfrey leaves, shredded

5 drops lavender oil

This will make about 6 bath bag inserts

Intensive Care Skin Softening Potpourri

½ cup chamomile flowers

½ cup yarrow flowers

½ cup oatmeal

½ cup lavender buds

¼ cup dry powdered milk

4 drops rose oil or rose geranium oil

This will make about 8 bath sachets.

Relaxing Bath Potpourri

½ cup catnip

½ cup sandalwood

½ cup bergamot

½ cup chamomile flowers

¼ cup dry powdered milk

3 drops bergamot oil

4 drops sandalwood oil

This will make about 8 bath sachets

Invigorating Bath Potpourri No 1

¼ cup rosemary

¼ cup pepperment leaves

¼ cup basil

8 bay leaves

¼ cup oatmeal

2 tablespoons whole cloves

This makes about 8 bath sachets

Invigorating Bath Sachet No 2

¼ cup sage

¼ cup rosemary

¼ cup spearmint

¼ cup sea salt

This makes about 6 to 8 bath sachets

Make your own bath sachet combinations using one or more of the herbs below with their corresponding essential oils.

Healing Herbs—Calendula, catnip, comfrey, dock, eucalyptus, lady's mantle, mint, oregano, raspberry leaves, sandalwood, sage

Stimulating Herbs—Basil, bay, calendula, fennel, lavender, lemon verbena, marjoram, mint, rosemary, sage, savory, thyme

Relaxing Herbs—Catnip, chamomile, comfrey, lavender, jasmine, lemon balm, rose, tansy, valerian, vervain

Magical Sachets

Magical sachets can be made to attract love, money, and success, to make one feel beautiful, and to heal and to protect one's self or home. The best material to use for these sachets is felt, silk, or another tight-woven fabric since the scent of the filling is unimportant. It is important to note that magical sachets should always be used for the good of a situation. They should never be made with the intent to do harm or to negatively influence someone. While making the sachet and the sachet fill one should always be mindful of the reason you are making it. Energize your materials with your intent. Seal them with knots woven into the ribbon.

To make a magical sachet follow the same procedure as making a scented sachet. These can be made larger or smaller as the need may be. Many colors are said to induce certain results. It would be advantageous to use colors for the effects desired. Below is listed the correct color for the desired results. Make sure your fabric and ribbon match or you can always use white cloth or ribbon for any situation.

Wealth, Prosperity, and Success—Green, gold, brown

Healing—Blue, black, orange

Beauty—Pink, magenta

Love—Pink, red

Protection sachets should be made with white cloth, denoting purity of thought. Tie with a red ribbon. To protect a house, hang from the highest point of the house. If this is impossible, hang over the main entrance or place a sachet in the corners of a room. If protecting a vehicle, place a sachet under the driver's seat. If protecting a loved one or yourself make sure it is carried on the person at all times. Fill protection sachets with a mixture of the following. Use equal parts of some or all:

Aloe—Include an aloe leaf in house sachets to be hung above the main entrance. This will guard the house against evil and household accidents.

Basil—Place a basil sachet in every room to protect the house and its occupants from evil.

Bay—Add to house protection sachets or carry a sachet with you to protect yourself from harm.

Dill—This is another house protection herb. Place in a sachet and hang over the door.

Fenne—Place both the leaves and seeds of this herb in a sachet to protect the home.

Garlic—Place an unpeeled clove of garlic in a sachet to protect those who will be traveling by water. Garlic powder or cloves of garlic in a house sachet will protect the house from evil and it will also protect the occupants from envious people.

Horehound—Place this in a sachet and hang over the doors or windows to protect house and occupants from sorcery.

Marjoram—Place in a house protection sachet.

Rosemary—Sachets of rosemary should be hung over doors to protect the house from thieves.

Sage—Place in a household protection sachet.

Saint John's Wort—Place a sachet containing this herb near windows to protect the house from lightening, fire and evil spirits.

Valerian—This herb protects the house from lightning.

Vervain—This herb also protects the house from lightning.

Be sure to mix all potpourri mixtures in a non-metal container. Earthenware is the best in which to concoct your fillers.

Wealth, prosperity, and success sachets can be filled with equal parts of some or all of the following:

Basil—Carry a basil sachet in the pocket, in a wallet, or in a purse to attract money. Place over the door of a business or inside the money box or cash register. You will have a successful business.

Chamomile—Carry with you or place over the door to attract money to you.

Mint—Carry a mint sachet with you at all times to attract money, and success.

Sage—Sage sachets will ensure that no one in your house is ever hungry and will guard against poverty when placed in the highest point of the house or over all entrances.

Woodruff—A sachet of woodruff should be carried with you to attract money.

Include acorns and orange peel with any of the herbs above in the sachets. These too attract success and prosperity.

To make a healing sachet fill combine the some or all of the following:

Coriander Seeds—Keep a sachet of seeds if you have recurring headaches. This will prevent them.

Eucalyptus—Keep a sachet with you to protect against colds or to ease one.

Hops—Carrying a hops sachet ensures good health

Lavender—Carrying this sachet or hanging it in a house ensures good health for all that live there.

Mint—Make a wrist sachet. Measure your wrist and make two strips 1½" wide and ½" shorter than the measurement for your wrist. Place ribbon on in the ends and sew within the seam. Sew all the way around leaving a small slit in which you can insert a funnel. Fill the sachet with mint. Don't fill too full because you want it to lie flat. Sew up the slit by hand. Now tie the sachet around your wrist by tying the ribbon together. This will ensure you will never be ill.

Rosemary—A sachet will promote healing

Sorrel—A sachet carried with you will protect the heart and helps wounds heal.

To make a sachet that will make you more confident and beautiful, mix some or all of the following and carry it in your pocket or put it in your bra:

Rose petals—Just the scent will make you feel more appealing.

Lavender—A sachet of lavender will make you absolutely irresistible.

Rosemary—Fill a sachet with rosemary and feel confident in what ever you do.

Jasmine—A jasmine sachet will also make you irresistible and charming.

To make a sachet to attract a lover, mix some or all of the following:

Lemon balm—Give a sachet of lemon balm to the person you wish to attract.

Basil—The scent of this sachet will attract a lover to you. Make sure they can smell it.

Bay—Add a bay leaf to a sachet to attract a man.

Catnip with Rose petals—Hold a sachet filled with these ingredients in your hand until it is warm then give to a prospective lover. They will be sure to follow you anywhere.

Cinnamon—Add this to a sachet to attract a woman.

Lavender—A lavender sachet is sure to entice a man.

Yarrow—Give a sachet of yarrow to the object of your desire and see what happens.

Give your scented and bath sachets to people for gifts. Scented sachets can be tied on the outside of a package instead of bows. Give a bath sachet with several types of bath potpourri. Use protection sachets for house warmings or wealth and prosperity sachets for weddings. The scented and bath sachets will be appreciated for their usefulness, while the magical sachets will be appreciated for the thought. Let each sachet work its magic in its own way.

Crafting Sweet Dreams

❧ By Carly Wall, C.A. ❧

O nce called comfort pillows, dream pillows have been used through the ages to soothe troubled sleepers through the gentle and restful aroma of the herbs stuffed inside of them. As a person tosses and turns restlessly, the herbs are crushed and so exude their scent; of course, care is taken only to choose the most rest-inducing herbs in a dream pillow.

Historically, herb pillows, which have been used since Biblical times, were also filled with such herbs as mandrake, which, when placed under a loved one's pillow, would ward off evil spirits. In centuries past, herb pillows of mugwort were reputed to induce dreams of one's future lover. Even in Native American culture, dream pillows were used medicinally, and for religious purposes. The medicinal

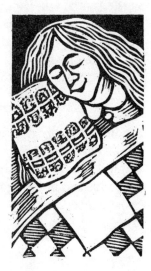

usage of herbal pillows was popular in medieval times, as monks would craft them to help soothe the sick in their sickrooms. They were used to help heal congested lungs, and to ease stressed patients worried about dying of the plague.

Today, you might imagine herbal pillows relegated to the role of decoration, since when we talk about them, often what comes to mind are the decorative little silk fluff pillows covered in lace and ribbon. Actually, nowdays herb pillows function in both ways. They can decorate a bedroom, guest room, or add charm to a characterless couch, and yet they have the attractive quality of being really useful.

The Quality of Herbs

Certain herbs have aromatic qualities that really affect our senses and our psyche. This fact falls between the realm of herbalism and aromatherapy. The aromatic molecules of herbs are inhaled and sent directly to the limbic portion of the brain— which is the seat of our emotions, sexuality, creativity, and imagination. Scent really does have a powerful physiological effects on our bodies and minds. If you want to test this, merely purchase some pure and natural lavender essential oil, and clary sage essential oil. Place a few drops on a light bulb ring, light the lamp, and observe what effect the scent has on a room full of people. In no time at all, you should see people getting quieter and more drowsy, until, if the right conditions exist, some people may actually start to doze.

Herbs and Dreams

Studies have proven that dreaming is essential for a healthy mind. Dream images and actions are the subconscious mind's way of communicating with the conscious, of working out problems and pointing the way to solutions, of entertaining and enhancing creativity.

In a stress-filled world we can still use dream pillows to find ever-elusive comfortable sleep. The effect of herbal aroma is not only quite strong on the subconscious mind—thus quickly inducing sleep— but this much more gentle on the body than the effect of sleeping pills. Dream pillows work quite well with children too, aiding in chasing away nightmares, calming restlessness, helping ease and comfort in times of sickness. And herbs are, of course, much safer for children.

It's really very easy to create wonderful little dream pillows for yourself, your family, and your friends. The first step is simple—deciding which herb or herbs you want to add to a pillow to achieve particular results. And from there you just have to create the pillows to add the herbs to. To begin, you should be aware of the different effects that specific herbs have. Here are a list of herbs and their effects, and some suggested combinations of herbs you can choose from when making your pillows. Make sure you take great care with certain herbs, or you may cause effects you never intended.

Herbs for Restless Dreams

Russian tarragon—frightening dreams

Sage—creates a lost feeling or sense of imprisonment in dreams

Tansy—violent and terrifying dreams and also headaches when awakening

Herbs for Peaceful Dreams

Aniseed (Pimpinella anisum)—this fragrance is relaxing and has the odd ability to inhibit men from dreaming when they need to cease thinking about things.

Balsam fir (Abies balsamea)—pleasant and refreshing fragrance. Good for when you have respiratory problems or colds.

Catnip (Nepeta cataria)—Use sparingly to help send off to restful sleep. Eases babies' sleep.

Chamomile (Chamaemelum nobile)—good for children and elderly. Soothing, good for insomnia and bad dreams. Sweetly scented.

Cinnamon (Cinnamomum zeylanicum)—proven to bring on erotic dreams for men. An exotic addition to the dream pillow.

Clary Sage (Salvia sclarea)—sleep-inducing, and helpful with depression and stress. Proven to create a balance in calming tension and taking away fatigue. It helps to deepen the breath and opens the chest from a tight, constricted feeling. Especially effective when combined with eucalyptus and pine for coughs, throat infections, and bronchitis. If you've been moody, indecisive, and confused, this is one to add to the blend. It allows inspiration to flow.

Clove (Syzygium aromaticum)—Adds a refreshing spiciness to the blends.

Frankincense (Boswellia carterii)—this is a resin which comes from a small tree that is steam-distilled to make an essential oil. It deepens the breath, is anti-infectious and very soothing. Helps energy to flow and is tranquillizing. Stills the mind and causes the spirits to soar. Takes away stress and bad feelings. If you have been oppressed or weighed down by heavy thoughts, add a few drops to your blend.

Hops (Humulus lupulus)—the flower from a perennial vine. Helps soothe to sleep.

Jasmine (Jasminum officinale)—induces exotic and romantic dreams for women.

Lavender (Lavandula spp.)—eases headaches, relaxing. Adds warmth, feelings of safety. Lavender scent cools and calms. It encourages full expression of creativity.

Lemon balm (Melissa officinalis)—relieves depression, insomnia, tension, and anxiety.

Lemongrass (Cymbopogon citratus)—soothes and creates an exotic feeling in dreams.

Lemon verbena (Aloysia triphylla)—makes you fly in your dreams.

Marjoram, sweet (Origanum majorana)—eases nervousness and restlessness during sleep.

Mint (Mentha spp.)—adds clarity, color and vivid images to dreams.

Mugwort (Artemisia vulgaris)—it is said this herbs helps one remember dreams. It also is said to increase clarity and at the same time promote relaxation and soothing, calming feelins.

Rose (Rosa spp.)—loving thoughts and peaceful dreams. Helps in easing grief.

Rosemary (Rosmarinum officinalis)—used down through the ages to chase away nightmares and ensure good sleep. Works well with lavender, roses, mugwort, hops. Deters remarkable dreams. Helps concentration, lethargy, strain, emotional exhaustion.

Thyme (Thymus spp.)—encourages dreams of creativity and flight, and was once thought to allow a dreamer to see fairies. Good for any weakness or congestion of the lungs. It is an expectorant, antiseptic, and tonic. Helps depressive states which have to do with withdrawal, pessimism, and self-doubt.

Blending Herbs

Use a combination of dried herbs in equal amounts according to the effects you want to achieve from the scents. You may choose also to enhance scents by adding several drops of essential oils (not too much, you don't want to overwhelm the senses!) to the dried herbs. You may also just want to use a select herb or two—in the past I've had good results simply using rose petals or lavender buds in a pillow.

Mix the herbs well, place the mixture in a sealed plastic bag for 24 hours to let the scents blend. After you've crafted your dream pillow and placed the herbs inside, make sure to store the pillow during the day in a plastic bag so that the freshness of the scents is assured. You can use the dream pillows up to two weeks before you must renew your herbs.

Creating Your Dream Pillow

How simple or complex you want to make your dream pillow is up to you. In Victorian times, the pillows were fancy, made with silk fabrics and lace. For quick dream pillows, you can use cotton handkerchiefs by placing the herbs in middle, gathering the ends of the cloth, and tying it with string. For our purposes, we'll create an actual little cloth "pillow" you can adapt to your sensibilities—whether fancy or plain—as you wish.

To start, choose a decorative piece of fabric about five by twelve inches in size—cotton is probably the best cloth due to its "breathable" qualities. Fold the cloth in half, inside out. You now have a five by six inch size of (folded) fabric. Stitch up three sides and turn right side out. Fill this with one-half to one cup of your dream blend, and sprinkle a few drops of an essential oil of choice. Fold down the open end and stitch this closed. Add decorative lace or ribbon as you please.

After you've created your pillow and filled it with your herbal blend of choice, you then tuck it inside your pillowcase at night for a good night's restful sleep.

Sample Blends

Peaceful Sleep

When you've been worrying yourself silly, use this blend to relax and sleep comfortably.

½ cup mugwort

½ cup lavender flowers

½ cup rosemary

3 to 4 drops lavender essential oil

Congested Chest

1 tablespoon each:

catnip

mugwort

peppermint

marjoram

Add several drops eucalyptus essential oil or frankincense.

Soothing Dreams

When you want to just get away from the world, use this blend to create new worlds of your own.

½ cup chamomile

½ cup mint

½ cup rose petals

Add a few drops of chamomile essential oil or clary sage. To make exotic dreams, add one of the spices—-cinnamon or clove.

Romantic Dreams

This blend is a good way of letting all those pent-up passions out!

   4 whole cloves

   1 Tablespoon mint

   1 cinnamon stick

   ½ cup rosemary

   ½ cup lavender

   ½ cup rose petals

Add a few drops of jasmine essential oil.

Creative Dreams

When you are having trouble with a particular project or have had trouble coming up with a solution to a problem, this blend will help you dream up the solution.

   ½ cup lemon verbena

   ½ cup rosemary

   ½ cup clary sage

   ½ cup hops

Add a few drops of frankincense essential oil.

Herb
History,
Myth, and
Magic

A Witch's Herbal Primer

By Silver Sage

Centuries ago herbs were used for more than just seasoning soup. In fact, herbs were not used as seasoning much at all.

But Witches—the Wise Ones, the ancients—they knew the magical uses of herbs. They used herbs in potions, incenses, and amulets in order to ward off evil, attract prosperity, protect a child, and heal illnesses. Much of this lore was forgotten, but fortunately for our contemporary generations, not all of it has been lost. Because of today's awareness of Earth's fragility, modern Wiccans, Pagans, and Witches are once again focusing on the gifts that the Mother has given us.

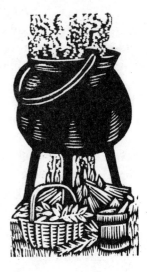

But just what is magic? Most of us are familiar with the Houdini style of prestidigitation, sleight-of-hand, illusion, stage-type magic. To Witches and Pagans, however—as one might guess—magic is much more than an illusory stage trick. Magic is the influencing of the environment by using the natural energy that surrounds us.

Just as our minds and our bodies work together and influence each other, the physical and psychic (or astral) planes are also linked. The astral can influence the physical as easily as the physical can the astral; it all comes together in beauty, within the laws of nature.

There are many earth-oriented, goddess-oriented, Wiccan or Pagan religions that practice magic. However, magic is not necessarily a religious practice. Some traditions believe that magic should always be a religious rite, while there are other traditions that use magic as a tool for everyday living, giving it no religious implications at all. Whichever way you approach magic is equally valid. The purpose here is to discuss how herbs may be used in magical amulets, potions, rituals, and ceremonies.

Tradition has it that magic should only be worked for good. The three-fold law that many Wiccans and Pagans believe says that whatever you send out will come back three times over. So if you work magic for good, good will come back to you three times over! But remember the reverse holds true, if you work for harm to come to someone, well...

Supplies You May Need

In my magical practice, I have used ritually consecrated bollines and plain kitchen knives; I've used mortars and pestles, a pottery bowl, and the back of a spoon. In my opinion, it's not how fancy the tools are as long as they do the job. However, there are some things that will make magical practice a little easier or possibly more esthetically pleasing—certain tools you may eventually find indispensible. These include a mortar and pestle for grinding herbs, a knife for harvesting herbs, a non-metallic pot for brews, and a special basket or tray reserved for preparing herbs.

You can collect your own herbs, but many of us live in large cities and sprawling urban areas overrun by parking lots. Also, many herbs grow only in specific areas. You probably won't find mistletoe in the middle of the Mojave Desert, for example. Nor are you likely find chaparral in Ohio. In that case, you can use commercially dried herbs, as long as you are sure they are organic or wild-harvested. Chemical fertilizers, weed-killers, and pesticides can indeed ruin an otherwise wonderful herb.

Purchased herbs come in many forms, powdered, whole, or what is called "cut and sifted." I usually use herbs that are in chunks or pieces—the "cut and sifted" variety—preferring to imbue them with my own intent and energy during the grinding process. Some herbs, however, are very difficult to grind. Frankincense and myrrh, for instance are hard and resistant to hand grinding, and will gum things up as well. I usually purchase these two herbs already powdered.

If you are going to collect or grow your own, remember that traditionally among many Wiccans or Pagans, Samhain (October 31) is considered the day of final harvest. As such, it is the last date to gather herbs for use during the rest of the year. The reasoning behind this is that as the year progresses the plant's life force begins to wane. As the physical year progresses from fall to winter, plants tend to become apathetic, if not downright dormant. If you are going to use an herb in a spell, a ritual, or even in incense, you want it to be full of potent energy.

Plant energy is at its height from late spring to late summer. Gathering herbs at that time pretty much assures that the dried plant has lots of life-force left for you to call on when necessary. Two or three cuttings a season are usually possible from a properly cared for garden, or even in the wild. If you are harvesting in the wild, be sure to stay at least thirty yards from the roadway, pay attention to any possible sources of toxins or pollutants, and only take a tenth of the plant to assure its survival so that you can harvest again.

Herbs, like candles, colors, and many other things in magic and ritual practice, have correspondences. I've heard people say that it doesn't matter a bit if the herb is masculine or feminine, whether its element is fire or water, they just use it however they want. "It's the intent that's important." It's true, intent is very important, and if that approach works for you fine, but intent is simply not the only factor at work in magic.

I like to consider carefully each herb that I'm using, and to work hard so that the herbs I use won't cancel each other out. My advice is pay attention to the correspondences of herbs, as well as the moon phases when they will be most effective. If you don't have an emergency situation, take the time to carefully plan your ritual or spell. Look up the best planetary hours or at least the correct day. If you are using candles or other accessories, consider color correspondences as well! Careful planning usually translates into a much more effective spell.

Herbal House Cleansing and Protection Ritual

Ever felt a sensation that something just wasn't right—your house didn't seem like home anymore, or a visitor left bad energy behind them? Perhaps a purification rite is in order. If you combine a few select herbs you can cleanse and protect your home. In fact, There are many herbs with purifying properties: Bay, mugwort, yarrow, cedar, rosemary, sage, angelica, basil, lavender, elder, and juniper, just to name a few.

Let us put a few of these together, balancing their attributes for a good purifying and protective mix. Cedar, bay, and rosemary would be wonderful choices. They are masculine; as children of the sun their element is fire. They are perfect for spiritually protecting and purifying your home.

Lavender would add a little air to the mix, helping the herbs burn well, and as a masculine herb would complement the strength and positive energy of the others. Daughter of earth, vervain is important for her grounding qualities; she will purify and protect the house on a mundane level. And lastly, elder is a very strongly protective herb that, with its associations to the feminine and to water, will maintain the equilibrium.

You'll need about a cup of dried herbs, as well as several four to six inch branches of rosemary or bay, if available. Place the leaves and stems into a bowl or cup, and pour boiling water (about two cups) over the herbs. Cover to keep the volatile oils from escaping and let it steep for at least thirty minutes. Strain.

The best day for protection magic is probably Saturday. Monday also is beneficial to household matters. The waxing Moon is favorable if you want to increase the purification results and the protective effects. If it's not too cold, open the windows and doors to your home. Think about the cleansing effects that are your goal. Visualize the strengths of the herbs you are using as you take advantage of their various properties to protect your home. Consider the power that is in everything around you, the energy that is there for you to use. Tap into this power and feel the increased sensations as you gather this energy to you. Call on your deity to aid and ensure the success of your endeavor. Start in the east, and using a branch of rosemary as an aspergill, move deosil (sunwise) around your entire house, sprinkling as you go. If you don't have access to the small branches of rosemary, just use your fingers to sprinkle!

As you face the east, beckon the powers of air. Feel its purifying breath as it whispers through your home, feel the positive energy collecting and taking the place of the negativity. In the south, call to the element of fire. Feel its warmth; feel it burning away all the darkness has taken residence. Visualize light in every corner, sparkles dancing in the sunbeams. The west is the place of renewal. Call gently on the forces of water, picturing the waves of rebirth washing through your home, cleansing every little corner, crack, and crevice. In the north you will summon earth with all its strengths. Envision the earth absorbing the negativity, and see earth-power collecting in abundance to protect you and yours. Return to the east, closing the circle.

The next step is to cense the house with rosemary incense. Light one of the remaining branches, and walk the same circuit you did before, seeing the fragrant smoke from the rosemary gathering anything dark and whisking it away into the cosmos. Carefully, draw a protective pentagram in the air at each window and door with the smoldering branch. If no branches are available, sprinkling crushed dried rosemary leaves on a charcoal disk works just fine, and the pentagram can be drawn in the air with your hand. When you're finished, close the windows and doors, and say a sincere "blessed be."

Healing Spell

A friend is sick, been to the doctor, and is taking what's been prescribed. But they need some spiritual uplifing—a bit of magic to boost the energies. The following is very easy to do while you are visiting a sick friend.

To begin, mix an incense of one part rosemary and one part juniper. Burn this in tiny quantities in the sick room, and visualize the illness being wafted out of the patient and into the ether along with the smoke of the incense. Mix the following powders together: two parts eucalyptus, one part myrrh, one part thyme, and one part allspice. Sprinkle this powder around the room as you recite the following chant:

> The Goddess walks before (patient's name), and sees that she/he is suffering with (here list the condition or symptoms). She speaks and says "You will be healed, you will be healed, you will be healed." It is done. In the name of the maiden, mother, and crone, blessed be. We who believe in the Goddess she blesses with these signs: We shall speak with love, we shall drive out all negativity, we will not be harmed by ill-intentions. Our hands shall be extended to the sick and they soon will be healed. In the name of the maiden, mother, and crone, blessed be.

Repeat three times, visualizing the illness leaving the patient, and the patient arising whole and well. Adapted from *Hexcraft* by Silver RavenWolf.

Herbs and Candles

Herbs and candles have gone hand in hand for centuries. Incense and candles are very often combined in prayers, rituals, and religious ceremonies all over the world. Many incenses are made from herbs. Candles can be made with essential oils or have pieces of herbs incorporated into the wax. Herbs can be placed around the candle, under the candle, or the candle can be "dressed" with appropriate oils prior to burning.

Herb and Candle Spell for Monetary Abundance

Once again there's too much month left at the end of the money, and the dog needs his shots, the kids need new shoes, and the fridge is empty. What can you do to tide you over till payday? You could rob a bank, hit up your relatives, or, instead, you might employ a bit of magic.

On a Thursday, the best day for matters of material wealth, take out a green candle for money (or a blue one for material gain) and dress it with bergamot oil and orange oil. Orange is used for drawing money. Its elemental association is fire. Bergamot, also a money herb, has an elemental association to air which helps fuel the fire of orange. To dress the candle, combine a small amount of the two oils. Apply the oil to the candle from the tip to the center and from the bottom to the center. This is so you will attract the money. If you were trying to push something away, you would apply the oil from the center to the tip. As you are applying the oil, see money coming in from different sources; a bonus perhaps, a loan payback, or a refund of a deposit. You may want to inscribe a dollar amount, or just dollar signs into the candle, visualizing just enough money stuffing your purse or pocket to buy the shoes and fill the fridge. Next, hold the candle in your power hand. Ask for your deity's assistance in the success of the spell. Draw energy from the earth or from the universe around you and imbue the candle with energy, visualizing the realization of your goal.

You can put a pinch of vervain in the candleholder before you put the candle into the holder. The vervain is "to make it go" and to reinforce the financial attraction. You might sprinkle a bit of cinnamon around the base of the holder too, as cinnamon is traditionally considered to be a good money magnet.

If you choose, you could burn some ginger incense to increase the chances of success. In addition to ensuring the success of the spell, ginger also attracts money. Now, sit before the candle, ground and center, light the candle, and focus your mind on the flame. Meditate on the amount of money that you need, let visions of what you will do with your newfound funds flow through your mind. Smell the ginger and the orange as the candle burns, and let the scents sink into your consciousness knowing that they mean monetary gain. When the candle burns down completely, complete the spell by disposing of the leftover wax by burying it or casting it into a source of running water.

Charms and Amulets

Health

It's flu and cold season, and you can't seem to get away from the germs. A good magical remedy is to place a handful of coriander seeds into a green bag and tie it tightly. Invoke the energy and power of the four elements, and infuse the energy into the amulet—grounding any excess energy and carrying it with you. This simple amulet has been used to repel sickness for many years. And it certainly smells better than the garlic my great-grandmother wanted to tie around my neck to keep me healthy!

Protection

One of the simplest protective charms is to make a sachet using three protective herbs. Some of the herbs with protective qualities include: anise, bay, cedar, clove, dill, eucalyptus, frankincense, juniper, mugwort, myrrh, patchouli, sage vervain, and wormwood. Mix the three herbs that you have chosen together and place them in the center of a red or white piece of cloth. Gather the corners and tie them up. Charge the charm, saying words like "I charge you to guard and protect in the goddess' name." The charm should then be carried with you, placed it in the highest point of the house, under the driver's seat of the car, tied to your child's school bag, and so forth.

Another easy protective charm is also a very old one. Witches used to place an acorn in every room of the house for protection.

Group Protective Amulet

I recently made a group amulet to protect my mother, sister, and niece while they were travelling in Europe. The items I used for this charm were a cleansed purified quartz crystal, three sage leaves—one for each woman—some white, red, and black thread, and a small velvet bag. I went to the sage bed in the herb garden and selected big, healthy sage leaves. After writing the name of my mother, sister, and niece—one on each leaf—I wrapped them around the quartz crystal and secured the leaves to the crystal with white, red, and black thread signifying the maiden, mother, and crone. In addition, the three leaves, three women, and three colors of thread were symbolically sacred to the goddess. The leaf-wrapped crystal was then placed into a small black velvet bag. I blessed and consecrated the charm in the goddess' name for the purpose of protection, and then energized the charm. I decided to call earth energy since I wanted to protect my family from the mundane variety of thugs. Fortunately, I live near a large chunk of granite, so I grounded myself, extended my receiving hand, and called earth energy to me. I felt my skin tingle as it flowed into my body and went into the charm. When the charm felt full, I stopped the flow and grounded the excess. The charm was ready for its trip to Europe. When it returned, I placed the charm on my altar until I had a chance to disassemble it, cleanse the crystal, and place the leaves and the thread into the earth, grounding any energy that remained.

Herbal Correspondences for the Holidays

For Ostara, you may decorate your altar with figures of bunnies and freshly gathered spring flowers, and you should burn rose petals, lavender, and cinnamon as incense. These make a suitably cute and fresh-smelling ritual, but unfortunately they do not quite capture the energy of the season. Correspondence-wise, the herbs you use for incense, anointing oils, or to decorate your altar should bring the correct associations and energies for the Spring Equinox. With just a bit of research you can discover which are flowers of Venus and which plants belong to the Earth. You'll know what to put in your incenses, oils, or powders to tie your seasonal celebrations all together.

Remember, as you are choosing herbs to combine for esbats and sabbats, that you are really creating the mix to enhance what you are doing. It's not especially critical for the mix to smell good, though smelling good is always a bonus; smell is not the primary reason for mixing the herbs. When gathering herbs for an incense, be sure to include a resin. The resin binds the ingredients together and helps the incense burn. Match the resin as best you can to elemental or astrological correspondences. If that doesn't work, use the purpose of the herb. If you still can't find a match anywhere, then go for pleasing fragrance!

Herbs for an Esbat (Full Moon)

Any of the following are associated with the moon: camellia, coconut, cotton, gardenia, jasmine, lily, sandalwood, willow, wintergreen, lemon balm, eucalyptus, and myrrh. Decorate your Full Moon altar with white herbs such as sage, oak moss, and wormwood. White flowers on the altar for a Full Moon ritual are simply beautiful as the Moon illuminates the petals with an ethereal glow. Being white, gray, or silvery in color, their energies correspond quite nicely to the pale intensity of the moon.

Powder and mix equal parts of the following: sandalwood, myrrh, jasmine flowers, benzoin; and bless, consecrate, energize, and burn them as Full Moon incense.

Herbs and Plants for the Sabbats

There are a wide variety of correspondences that can be used when deciding which herbs and plants to use in your holiday celebrations. Most of us use pine and fir, holly and ivy for Yule, fresh flowers and eggs for Ostara, nuts, pumpkins, whole grain breads or muffins for Samhain and so on. In addition you may want to consider the Celtic Tree month associations when looking for appropriate altar decorations. These shift year to year, so the holidays don't always fall within the same Tree month. Best bet is to consult a magical type almanac for the correct tree.

Samhain (Air, Venus)—Samhain marks the new year for Pagans. Apples and pumpkins have long been a symbol of this season. It is thought that the Isle of Avalon (avalon meaning "apple") was where the body of King Arthur was taken and it got its name from the numerous apple trees that grew there. If you cut an apple in half crosswise, you'll see the five-pointed star that many Pagans consider a sacred symbol. Pile the altar high with apples. you can always munch the decorations if you get hungry. I've also used small pumpkins for my quarter candles on Samhain. Carve one side with runes representing something you wish to manifest in the coming year, and carve the appropriate elemental symbol into the other. It looks great from inside the circle or out. You can choose among the following herbs for your Samhain needs: Alder, anise, apple, balm of gilead, barley, bergamot, orange, cardamom, caraway, elder, fenugreek, geranium, hibiscus, hops, lavender, licorice, marjoram, mugwort, orris, pine, plumeria, raspberry, rose, wood sorrel, tansy, thyme, tonka, valerian, vanilla, vervain, and vetivert.

Samhain Incense

1 part gum acacia or Arabic (psychic powers)

1 part vetivert (to guard against hexes)

1 part lavender (to protection and attract love)

½ part mugwort (psychic powers)

Few drops of mugwort oil

Powder and mix thoroughly and burn during Samhain rituals to help "see" beyond the veil.

Yule (Winter solstice, Earth, Saturn)—The time of renewal, when the Sun god returns to bring warmth and fertility to the land. Pine cones and holly sprigs entwined with ivy, red and green candles anointed with a few drops of patchouli (for longevity and protection) can all be arranged on your altar for Yule. Alfalfa, bistort, barley, cypress, horsetail, honeysuckle, horehound, ivy, lobelia, magnolia, mugwort, patchouli, vervain, and vetivert all have Earth-Saturn correspondences and should be considered when planning your Yule celebrations.

Yule Powder

Alfalfa (to guard against poverty and hunger)

Vetivert (for prosperity and luck)

Ivy (for fidelity and love)

Grind equal parts fairly fine and sprinkle around the house at Yule or around the perimeter of the circle after it has been cast for the Yule sabbat celebrations.

Imbolc (Air, Saturn, Uranus)—At Imbolc we are celebrating the banishing of winter and welcoming the returning springtime. With more daylight hours, we know that spring is on its way, even as the snowflakes continue to pile up. Try some of the following herbs for your Imbolc activities: anise, benzoin, orange bergamot, cypress, dandelion, dock, hops, horsetail, ivy, lavender, lemon grass, mullein, mace, marjoram, mint, patchouli, pine, sage, skullcap, or southernwood. My own Imbolc celebration consists of invoking Brigid's presence (it's Brigid's Day as well, you know) as hearth-mother. Then I go through the house lighting candles dressed with lavender oil for peace and happiness in every room. Tradition has it that the candles should be lit in every window at sundown and left burning until sunrise. The plethora of brilliantly burning candles is reminiscent of the ancients kindling great fires on the tops of all the tors on this day. Next, briefly, I open a window or door in every room, symbolically inviting the freshness of the coming spring inside to dispel the darkness of winter. As I go through the house deosil I like to sprinkle some banishing powder to dispel winter gloom and brighten the energies around me.

Imbolc Banishing Powder

Benzoin (for purification and clearing)

Ivy (to guard against negativity

Lavender (to encourage happiness and peace

I use two parts lavender to one part ivy and one part benzoin. These should all be powdered or in fairly small pieces. Energize the powder with thoughts of clear spring days and dedicate it to the deity of your choice.

Ostara (Spring equinox)—I always look forward to change in season, but in spring, as the buds are suddenly bursting and as Mother Nature shows her abundance and fertility, I am always amazed! An altar decorated with pastel candles and ribbons, snapdragons and sunflowers or marigolds, and a bit of flowering sweet woodruff for a green accent is delightful. Ostara herbs are: allspice, basil, coriander, cedar, cinquefoil, ginger, high john the conqueror, marigold, peppermint, pine, rosemary, snapdragon and sweet woodruff.

Ostara Incense

Ginger (love and increase)

Coriander (love and health)

Peppermint (to excite love)

Dragon's Blood (for sexual potency)

Mix one part coriander, peppermint, and dragon's blood, and one-half parts Ginger, or adjust to your own preference. Grind all to a find powder and energize while visualizing abundance all around you. Ask blessings for a bountiful spring.

Beltaine (Earth, Venus)—The correspondences for Beltaine are Earth and Venus, so you can't find much better energy than this! Venus has long brought images of love to mind, and the throbbing heartbeat of the Earth always inspires as the God and Goddess come together to ensure the earth's continued fertility. My Beltaine altar is usually full of blooms and greenery such as apple blossoms, cypress, oleander, elder flower, and bunches of sweet pea. Herbs to consider for Beltaine are: apple, apricot, cypress, balm of gilead, barley, cardamom, catnip, elder, honeysuckle, oleander, patchouli, heather, geranium, hyacinth, lilac, mugwort, myrtle, passion flower, plumeria, sweet pea, tonka, and vanilla.

Anointing Oil for Beltaine

2 parts Plumeria

2 parts Vanilla

1 part Cardamom

Mix together and dilute with a bit of good quality vegetable oil (almond, apricot, jojoba). This will give you a flowery, romantic scent, with a hint of spice!

Litha (Water, Moon)—Summer has just begun, and it's the time of the Sun in all his power and glory. We also celebrate lust and passion, successful crops, and fertility in all its guises. Try some of these when planning your Summer Solstice activities: camellia, chamomile, columbine, feverfew, gardenia, jasmine, lemon balm, mimosa, lemon, lotus, myrrh, pansy, rose, strawberry, and sweet pea.

Summer Flower Water

Gather a selection of flowers from the above list; cover with pure water and simmer for several hours until the fragrance suits you. You may strain the flowers out and add more if you need to for more intense fragrance. Add water as needed. When sufficiently aromatic, strain out the flowers and put the water into a pretty glass container, adding a few fresh flowers to the water for ambiance, and sprinkle or spritz when a cooling breath is needed during the Midsummer festivities!

Lughnassadh (Fire, Sun)—This is the beginning of the harvest cycle, when a tomatoes right off the vine or a peach just off the tree taste wonderful. At Lughnassadh we also honor the Celtic God Lugh, whose sacrificial death and rebirth is represented by a sheaf of grain, which symbolizes that even a God must give homage to his Goddess through whose benevolence he is reborn. Sheaves of wheat or oats often adorn my altar to represent his sacrifice. There are lots of herbs and plants with fire and Sun correspondences, such as: acacia, allspice, ash, bay, cedar, cinquefoil, chamomile, chrysanthemum, cinnamon, clove, copal, frankincense, hawthorne, juniper, oak, olive, and rosemary.

Harvest Incense

Frankincense (drive out negativity)

Juniper (health)

Hawthorn (happiness)

Oak (prosperity)

Mabon (Air, Venus)—This is the time of year I love the most! The leaves are beginning to turn, the air is crisp, the sky is clear and blue. Mabon marks a new cycle—as the nights begin to get longer, the time of the Crone is beginning and the last of the harvest has been taken in.

Autumn Incense

Benzoin (for prosperity)

Thyme (for courage)

Linden (for immortality)

Hazel (for wishes)

Use equal parts of each herb. Grind into a powder and blend completely. When you energize think of your ancestors, and how they had to face mounting hardship as the days began to get shorter for the coming winter. Think of the great courage they required simply to cope with the approaching hard-times.

Prosperity was likely what your ancestors hoped for at this time, if only so they could survive the winter and so continue on the cycle of life. Think about what is needed for continuation of your life, what kind of courage you need in the upcoming months, and what exactly you wish for in the coming months.

Next time it's your turn to come up with the ritual incense or a new holiday celebration, don't forget the herbs and plants. They embody the four elements and spirit. Each plant is nurtured in the earth, warmed by the fire of the sun, slaked with rain and blessed by the air. The result is the ever-present spirit and life force that is that herb. With some thought and planning you can call on this precious energy to enhance you spells, rituals, and your very life.

Mushrooms and Toadstools

❧ By Eileen Holland ☙

Mushrooms and toadstools are fungi, not plants, but since some of them can be used like herbs they are sometimes included in herbals and can have a variety of uses.

In general, fungi thrive on moisture. They love heavy dew, rainy weather, and warm, humid conditions. They reproduce by spores, which mushrooms produce in the spongy gills under their caps. Some fungi feed on dead or decaying matter like fallen leaves or rotting logs, while others need living hosts like trees or grass.

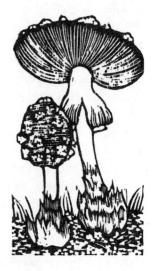

Mushrooms and toadstools, meanwhile, are actually the same thing—the fleshy "fruit" of fungi. Edible ones are usually called mushrooms, the inedible ones toadstools. Typically they resemble umbrellas, with a stem and a cap. They may also have a volva, a cup in the ground from which the stem rises.

Sometimes called death cups, these occur in both poisonous and non-poisonous varieties.

There are many kinds of fungi—yeast and mold included—but the fungi that concern us here are large net-like structures that can grow underground or in the wood of trees. When they get ready to reproduce they flower, shooting up spore-producing bodies, or mushrooms. Spores then are carried by water, wind, and animals, and when one lands in a hospitable place, a new fungus begins to grow from it.

Mushrooms provide protein, are very low in fat, and can help lower blood pressure. Popular culinary varieties include the common white button mushrooms that supermarkets carry, morels, chanterelles, enoki, porcini, shiitake, and oyster mushrooms. Not all mushrooms are edible, though. They were used as poison in ancient Rome, so Roman emperors would only eat those they had picked and prepared themselves. Mushrooms can be cultivated indoors in organic compost that has been treated with spores. They need to be kept at a constant temperature and free of drafts, humidity, and insects. Caves and windowless structures are popular places to grow mushrooms.

Mushroom Magic

Mushrooms and toadstools have always been considered agical because they appear overnight, seemingly out of nowhere, and sometimes disappear just as suddenly. There are many superstitions connected with them. For instance, mushrooms were thought to grow as the moon wanes—and in fact scientists now suspect that lunar cycles do affect their growth. In Japan, it was thought that thunder produced mushrooms and toadstools. Greeks and Aztecs believed they were engendered by lightning. Christians believed that mushrooms sprang up where St. Peter spat bread on the ground, and toadstools where the devil spat.

Mushrooms were considered unfit for human consumption in places where it was believed they were bad omens. Many Witches who are great cooks, and likely to have their own unique recipes for delicious mushroom dishes, also know that mushrooms can be used in magic. Mushrooms can be used for lunar magic, faery magic and water spells. Toadstools can be used in weather magic. Mushrooms correspond to the Moon, especially the Full Moon. Water is their element, and they have yin energy. In the animal kingdom toadstools correspond to reptiles, especially serpents. They have much in common with the skin of the toads for whom they are named, since there are varieties of both that produce exotic chemicals. Arabs call mushrooms Aish El-Ghorab (Raven's Bread).

Fairy Rings

Mushrooms and toadstools have long been associated with fairies, pixies, and other little people who are said to use them as stools and umbrellas. A fairy ring is a circle of toadstools that suddenly appears on a lawn. The grass within it is usually taller, darker, or brighter green than the rest of the lawn; there may be a patch of dead grass nearby. Because the rings appear seemingly by magic, some people believed they were caused by dancing fairies or elves, while others insisted they were caused by Witches, the fiery breath of dragons, or lightning strikes. They were also called fairy circles, fairy dances, hag's tracks and sorcerer's rings.

A fairy ring is a natural magic circle, a great place to cast a spell or make a wish, especially on the night of the Full Moon. Rings are said to have the power to bring good or bad luck, and cause or cure illness. You activate this power simply by stepping into them. A fairy ring in a field beside a house brings good fortune to the household. Harm was believed to come to a cow that stepped within a fairy circle or ate its grass. It was thought that you would become enchanted if you entered a ring during a Full Moon. Their dew was used to make love potions for young girls.

Fairy circles can live for hundreds of years. The rings grow outward, up to eight inches per year, as the fungus spreads underground. Thirty feet in diameter is their usual limit, but an large, 700-year old ring that stretched for miles was found in France.

If a pristine lawn is more important to you than a magic circle, you will find a fairy ring very hard to eradicate. The only sure way is to dig up the entire lawn to a depth of at least eighteen inches and resod the area. Marasmius oreades is the small, leathery toadstool that tends to form fairy rings more often than any other type of fungi. It has firm flesh and a knobbed cap that grows to two inches across, varying in color from ivory to light brown.

Mythology

There have been many myths about mushrooms through the ages. Edible mushrooms were considered food for the gods in ancient Greece and Mexico. Ixion, a Greek king who dared to make advances to Hera, was condemned by Zeus to Underworld. Mushrooms were the ritual tinder for the fire wheel Ixion was chained to. When Sisyphus founded Corinth, he peopled it with men sprung up from mushrooms. Perseus founded Mycenae in the place where a mushroom sprang up and supplied him with water. Tlaloc, Lord of Lightning, was the Aztec mushroom and toadstool god. Mushrooms were called Teonanacatl (Flesh of the Gods) in Central America, and there was a mushroom cult in ancient Mexico and Guatemala dating back to at least 1000 b.c.

Recipes

Stuffed mushrooms are a great appetizer I often make for parties and at Thanksgiving. Adjust quantities according to how many people you are feeding.

Seasoned bread crumbs

Grated parmesan or romano cheese

One tablespoon melted butter

One pound large white button mushrooms, cleaned and
    with their stems removed

Grated mozzarella cheese

Chicken or vegetable broth

Mix equal amounts of bread and cheese together. Add butter—you may have to add more to keep the mixture together. Turn the mushroom caps upside down in a glass baking dish. Mound the center of each one with the mixture, and press mozzarella cheese on top. Add enough chicken broth to cover the bottom of the pan about half way up the mushrooms. Cover the pan with aluminum foil and bake it in a hot oven (400°). Check it when the broth begins to bubble. If the mushrooms look baked, remove the foil and continue baking until the mozzarella melts atop each one. Cool slightly and serve. They look nice on a platter with cherry tomatoes.

Nectar of the Gods

Hallucinogenic mushrooms and toadstools have long been considered the nectar of the gods, imparting strange dreams and holy visions. They have been used in the religious rites of many cultures, ancient and modern. They were especially employed in the shamanic traditions of Siberia and the Americas, but also by the European mystery cults in their sacred rituals.

Magic Musrooms

Amanita muscaria—This toadstool is known as fly agaric, flycap, spotted toadstool, lighning mushroom, soma, asumer, and pong. Its Aryan name was Amrita, and its Siberian name Pongo. This white-spotted toadstool is the most famous sacred toadstool. It grows to twelve inches tall, the cap to fourteen inches wide. The older the toadstool, the more open its "umbrella." These spotted toadstools have white gills, white or yellowish stems, and tufted sides that emerge from a whitish death cup. Their flesh is firm and white. It was called flycap and fly agaric because a decoction of it was used to kill flies. Caution: Amanita muscaria is extremely poisonous. Overdose is lethal. Amanita muscaria is a psychedelic that acts on the central nervous system causing hallucinations, dizziness, and finally sleep. It can induce twilight sleep, producing a drowsy state with dream fantasies. It can also cause vomiting, vertigo, twitching, nausea, numbness, and death. Atropine is an emergency antidote.

Amanita toadstools are usually sliced, dried, then swallowed whole for ritual use. Siberian tribes drank the water in which the toadstools had been boiled. Those not invited to partake would drink the urine of those who had, because the drug passes whole out of the body that way. Yellow snow made by reindeer who had fed on the toadstools was eaten for the same reason. Amanita muscaria was introduced into India by Aryan peoples, who gathered it during the Full Moon and used it to make an intoxicating drink for religious rites. A spiritual food, it was called soma in India, haoma in Persia, and amrita in some Buddhist traditions

According to Robert Graves, the ingestion of amanita as ambrosia was part of the Orphic, Eleusinian, and other mystery cults. Amanita was sacred to Dionysus and his main intoxicant, supplying muscular strength for his revels. Centaurs (horse-totem tribespeople), satyrs (goat-totem tribespeople) and Maenads (the wild women), all associated with Dionysus, ate spotted toadstools to give themselves muscular strength and erotic power. In Koryak mythology, fly agaric sprang up wherever the god Vahiyinin (Existence) spat, as small white wapaq spirits with red hats. Vahiyinin advised Big Raven to eat the wapaq spirits when he needed strength. Big Raven was a culture hero who taught his people how to use the sacred toadstools. Viking warriors ate Amanita muscaria to give them their crazy power in battle. Some say Thor's hammer was a symbol of this toadstool. Native American tribes such as the Ojibwe also held it sacred and used it in their rites. Guatemalans called it the lightning mushroom, connected it with their storm god. A medieval fresco in Indres, France depicts a large amanita mushroom as the Tree of Knowledge, flanked by Eve and Adam, with the serpent wrapped around it. Some authorities hold that the Book of Revelation was written under its influence.

Amanita muscaria affects the psychic body, has been used by mages, yogis, shamans, and adepts of other paths in many ways:

for mystical experiences, in potions and libations, for spiritual evolution, to reach higher planes of consciousness, to induce ecstatic states, in fire rituals, to dissolve the ego and expand the consciousness. The toadstool itself is a charm for good luck. Amanita can be used charms and spells for fertility, happiness, health, wealth, good fortune, immortality, eternal youth and perfection. In some places, agaric found on old birch trees were added to the Beltane fire. The ashes of such a fire were a charm against witchcraft and malignant diseases of cattle and humans.

Death Cap

Amanita phalloides—This toadstool is known as death cup and deadly agaric; it is a deadly toxin. It contains the poison toxalbumin, which acts like rattlesnake venom. It destroys the liver and kidneys, dissolves red corpuscles, and causes the blood to drain out through the alimentary canal. In six to twenty-four hours after ingestion, cholera-like symptoms appear. Death occurs in three to five days—after intense suffering. Death cap, in fact, is so toxic that poisoning can occur simply by handling it or breathing its spores. Kidney dialysis and organ transplants are recommended treatments when the poisoning is quickly diagnosed.

Death Cap is a toadstool that varies in color from white to olive to brown. It has white gills and a ringed stem, and resembles edible mushrooms. It is often found in oak woods.

Destroying Angel

Amanita virosa—This toadstool contains deadly toxins. It is a white toadstool that grows to twelve inches and is found in pine and birch woods in the northern hemisphere.

Panther Cap

Amanita pantherina—a poisonous mushroom common in the Pacific Northwest. They are usually found under oak, pine, and fir trees, and may be discovered alone or in groups, in fall and spring. They have firm white flesh and round caps that range in color from dull yellow to dark brown, and grow from two to six inches in diameter on stems that can reach six inches high. The caps may have darker colored edges. Very young panther caps are covered by a whitish veil that turns into spots on the surface of the cap as the mushroom matures.

Dung Mushroom

Paneolus papilionaceus—This is a small, slender mushroom that contains a chemical that acts on the brain much like LSD. It is a mild hallucinogen with a mescaline-like effect. Dung mushrooms were used by Portuguese witches. They were considered the nectar of the gods, and may have been eaten by mystery cult adepts.

Psilocybe

Psilocybe are hallucinogenic North American and European toadstools found on grasslands and in alder woods. Mayans and other Native Americans used them to induce religious visions. Mayan priestesses invoked Tlaloc at the rites of the ingestion of the psilocybe mushrooms. European mystery cults may also have used them in their secret rites.

Magic Mushroom

Psilocybe baeocystitis—These are brownish or greenish, cone-shaped mushrooms. Magic mushrooms can be sticky from a thin film of jelly. Found from July until winter near evergreens on lawns, they grow to three inches and have no taste or smell. Their gills are almost entirely attached to the stem.

Liberty Cap, Liberty Bell Mushroom

Psilocybe semilanceata—Bell-shaped liberty cap mushrooms are common on grasslands and in tall grass beside roads and on golf courses. An ancient fresco depicts Demeter handing what looks like a liberty cap mushroom to Persephone, leading many to assume hallucinogenic mushrooms were part of the Eleusine mysteries.

Strophana

Psilocybe cyanescens—These are reddish-brown mushroom with dark gills and enlarged bases. They grow to four inches, have white flesh, and are found from July to September on lawns and in alder woods.

Elf's Stool

Psilocybe pelliculosa—This conical yellowish-green mushroom becomes sticky with a film of jelly when wet. Found in the debris of coniferous forests, it grows to three inches and has a musty odor.

Cultivator's Cap

Psilocybe strictipes—This toadstool contains the poison muscarine. Its caps are odorless yellowish-brown with straight stems. They have a thin film of jelly when wet, and are found from September to November in woods on conifers and rotting trees. They contain chemicals that affect the brain like LSD.

Psilocybe mexicana

This mushroom contains a hallucinogen that acts like LSD.

Other Interesting Fungi

Phallus impudicus (Stinkhorn, Common Stinkhorn, or Witch's Egg)—Stinkhorn is a phallus-shaped fungus with a spongy stalk that emerges from a round body, called the witch's egg, that lies half buried in the soil. Its cap leaks spores in a slimy fluid that smells like rotting flesh. Flies feed on the slime, spreading the spores. Stinkhorn is common in woodlands, usually found near rotting wood from late summer through the fall. It grows large in the tropics, and smaller in Europe and North America. Stinkhorn has been associated with witches and black magic. The egg-shaped structures it produces were once thought to be the eggs of evil spirits, and it was once used in used in love potions.

Claviceps purpurea (Ergot)—Ergot is a small purple fungus that grows as a parasite on cereal grasses such as rye. Ergot poisoning is characterized by convulsions and hallucinations. Some historians think that ergot poisoning, in the form of infected rye bread, was responsible for the delusions that led to the Salem witch trials. Grain poisoned by ergot was responsible for the

St. Anthony's Fire epidemic in Europe during the Middle Ages. Drugs derived from ergot include ergotaxine, used to stop uterine bleeding, and ergotamine, which was used to treat migraines. The psychedelic drug LSD can be made from ergot.

Lycoperdon bovida (Puffball)—A puffball is a rounded white fungus with thin skin that can grow to over eight inches. It is found under trees and on damp hillsides. Mature puffballs release black, powdery spores through a top vent when they are disturbed. Powdered puffballs are an astringent, and were used on cuts and wounds to control bleeding. Infusion or tincture of puffballs can be used to treat bleeding hemorrhoids.

Tuber magnatum (White truffle), and Tuber melanosporum: (Black truffle)—Truffles are rare fungi of two types, black and white, that grow entirely underground. They are found in Europe and the Pacific Northwest under trees, with which they have established a symbiotic relationship. Mature truffles have a strong smell that makes them prized by gourmets, but their scarcity makes them very expensive. Pigs and dogs are traditionally used to locate and unearth truffles.

Author's Caution: Never eat mushrooms you find growing wild. Many poisonous varieties look exactly like edible ones. Some will just make you very sick, but others will kill you in gruesome ways, so don't chance it. Do not ingest hallucinogenic fungi. They can kill you. There are far less dangerous ways to shapeshift, learn about past lives, open your third eye, or do astral projection.

Magical Mandrake

⇜ By Gerina Dunwich ⇝

*T*he mandrake is a poisonous narcotic plant associated with medieval Witchcraft and sorcery. It is also believed to be the most magical of all plants and herbs. Ruled by the planet Venus, it is potent in all forms of enchantment.

Mandrake, whose botanical name is Mandragora officinarum, is a native of the Mediterranean region. Its name means "man-dragon." A close relative to the nightshade family, it has purplish or greenish-yellow flowers, berries that seem to glow phosphorescently at sunrise, and a thick root that resembles the human body or a phallus. The flowers of this stemless perennial herb possess an unpleasant smell, and from its root a narcotic was formerly prepared. In the ancient Greek and Roman times, the juice of the root was used medicinally as an anesthetic prior to surgery and cauterization.

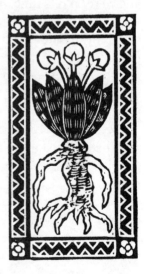

Caution should always be exercised when using any part of the mandrake in potions, brews, and philtres. It is a highly toxic plant, and misuse of it can result in sickness, delirium, or a slow and agonizing death. Authentic European mandrake is difficult to find in North America and quite expensive to buy. The "mandrake" sold at many occult supply stores and herbal shops in the United States is actually a plant called the mayapple (Podophyllum peltatum), which is a native of North America and in no way related to the European mandrake. The mayapple (or "American mandrake," as it is often called) possesses a single, nodding white flower and oval yellow fruit. Although the pulp of the ripe fruit is edible, the roots, leaves, and seeds of the "American mandrake" are just as deadly as its European counterpart.

It is said that there are female mandrake roots in addition to male ones. The female ones are often called "woman-drakes" and are shaped like the body of a woman. Both are equally as powerful in magic; however, many Witches of the female sex prefer to work with the female mandrakes, especially when spells dealing with love and sexuality are involved. In fact, mandrake root is the most powerful herb of love magic. Roots that resemble a phallus are believed to possess great aphrodisiac qualities and were, at one time, the main ingredient used in Witches' love philtres (potions) despite their highly toxic properties. According to Pliny the Elder, "When a mandrake root in the shape of a male genital organ was found, it secured genital love." In the Orient, mandrake roots are commonly sold in herbal shops and drugstores as a sex stimulant. They can be bought either whole or in powdered form, and usually at an exorbitant price.

A mandrake root soaked every Friday in a bowl of white wine and then carried in a charm bag made of red silk and velvet will give its possessor great sexual potency and attractiveness to the opposite sex. A mandrake root placed underneath a bed pillow will arouse passion between two lovers. In the Arab nations, many men who suffer from declining sexual potency wear a mandrake root on a necklace as a virility-enhancing amulet.

Female fertility is also promoted by eating mandrake (especially the female of the roots) or by carrying one as a charm, according to legend. (Editor's note: Don't do this!!) It has been used for centuries by women who desired large families and also by those who wanted to bear male children. In the book of Genesis, Joseph was said to have been conceived after Rachel, Jacob's wife, ate a mandrake root. According to folklore, the fruit of the mandrake can cause a man to fall in love with a woman if she gives it to him on Saint Agnes' Eve (January 20). A tiny particle of powdered female mandrake leaf added to a cup of red wine (for "passionate lovemaking") or white wine (for "romantic love") is said to be a powerful Witch's aphrodisiac.

In addition to love magic, mandrake roots are believed to possess the power to divine the future. More than one book on medieval Witchcraft and sorcery states that mandrake roots shake their heads to answer yes or no when questions are put to them. With the proper incantations, mandrakes can also be made to speak out. According to one "old wives' tale," if a mandrake root takes a liking to a novice magician, it will teach the novice certain highly sought-after secrets of the magical arts. Mandrake has been used by many modern Witches in spells and rituals that increase the psychic powers. They are carried in mojo bags or worn on necklaces as powerful charms to attract good luck.

In medieval times it was widely believed that special ointments containing powdered mandrake root were used by Witches. These ointments, which were called "sorcerer's grease," enabled Witches to fly, become invisible, or magically transform into animals and birds. Of course, Witches never did actually fly, become invisible, or shapeshift; however, the wild visions and sensations produced when the hallucinogenic ointments were absorbed into the skin more than likely led them to believe that they had.

In the country of Arabia, mandrake is called "Devil's candle" or "Devil's light." These nicknames derive from the folk belief that the plant's leaves glow in the dark, a phenomenon produced by glowworms, according to one source. The mandrake has, over the centuries and in various parts of the world, been given many other nicknames, including "man-dragon," "warlock root," "earth-manikin," "root of evil," and the "little gallows-man." The latter derives from the medieval legend that mandrake grows under a gallows tree from the blood of hanged criminals who were unbaptized. Mandrake roots should be uprooted from the earth only at night (especially when the Moon is Full), and always by the magician who intends to use it. Otherwise, the root's magical powers are useless. Another legend says that mandrake root shrinks whenever a man or woman approaches it, unless, of course, that person happens to be a Witch, a wizard, or someone who is in league with the Devil. Mandrake is one of the traditional ritual herbs of Samhain (Halloween), and is sacred to the following Pagan deities: Aphrodite, Diana, Hecate, and the legendary Teutonic sorceress known as the Alrauna Maiden.

Legend of the Screaming Mandrake

Medieval legend claims that when mandrake is uprooted, it emits an ear-piercing scream and begins to sweat blood. Legend also states that any man or woman who pulls the root from the earth is doomed to suffer an agonizing death. Many methods of safe mandrake harvesting were devised over the years by practitioners of sorcery and wizardry. The most popular method employed was to first loosen the soil around the mandrake plant with a shovel or other implement. Then, tie one end of a rope around a dog's neck and the other to the plant. The dog's master (who places cotton inside his ears to protect himself against the plant's deadly shriek) would then walk some distance away and command the dog to come to him. As the dog ran to its master, the root came up from the ground by the rope. The dog was killed by the evil scream, and the person was unharmed.

Circe's Plant

In Homer's second epic, the Odyssey, an enchantress by the name of Circe was said to have used a magical potion made from the juice of the mandrake root to inflame Odysseus' men with love and then turn them into swine. It was also from mandrake that she concocted a powerful magical poison that transformed the fair water-nymph Scylla into a grotesque and dangerous six-headed sea monster who destroyed everything that came within her reach. The ancient Greeks called the mandrake "Circe's plant" and dedicated it to this beautiful but deadly Witch goddess of the island of Aeaea.

Mandragoras

The term "mandragora" is used by herbalists for the narcotic prepared from the mandrake. At one time it was a word also used by poets to mean the entire mandrake plant. In folklore, mandragora is also a type of spirit or demon associated with mandrake. These supernatural beings are said to take the form of tiny, beardless men with black-colored skin. They roam secretly among the human population, causing mischief, and are summoned by sorcerers, whom they assist in the practice of black magic. Some mandragoras inhabit the roots of mandrake plants when not busy aiding magicians or amusing themselves by wreaking havoc on humans. Some mandragoras transform themselves into mandrakes, and others remain invisible but can be conjured with a special incantation recited over a mandrake root.

Curiously, while these spirits or demons are capable of inhabiting or changing into a mandrake root of either sex, the mandragora always remains of the male gender. Belief in mandragoras and their magical powers was common in Germany and Arabia throughout the Middle Ages. Many believed that these strange beings could bring madness to any man or beast if that was the will of the sorcerer who conjured them. Numerous charms and amulets were employed for protection against them. During the European Witch hunts, mandragoras were believed to have been the imps or demon familiars of Witches and warlocks. A mandrake root in one's possession was certain proof of sorcery to Witch-hunters.

Growing Your Own Mandrake

For a bit of homegrown magic, try planting a Witch's mandrake garden, or add this mystical plant to an existing herb or flower garden in your backyard. Mandrake can also be grown indoors in a flowerpot large enough to accommodate a foot-tall plant. Keep it near a sunny window (preferably one with a southern exposure), talk to it often, and give it some water once or twice a week.

European mandrake, which is propagated by seed or root division, should be planted in the center of small mounds of soil about twelve inches apart. Zone Seven of the United States Department of Agriculture's plant hardiness zone map (average minimum temperature of 0 to 10 degrees Fahrenheit) is the ideal climate for mandrake. Like most perennial plants, mandrake prefers full sunshine or partial shade, good soil, and proper drainage. Seed planting or root division should be done in early spring and when the Moon is full and/or in the astrological sign of Taurus, Capricorn, Pisces, Cancer, Scorpio, or Libra. Do not plant when the Moon is in its waning phase or in one of the barren signs: Leo, Gemini, Virgo, Sagittarius, Aquarius, or Aries.

In late spring, the mandrake blooms with greenish-yellow flowers that grow in the shape of bells, approximately one inch long. Its leaves have a wrinkled appearance and grow to be about twelve inches in length. The mandrake is not considered to be an ornamental plant, and in days of old it was grown only in the medicinal garden by folk healers and Witches who used its root as a painkiller and a sedative.

I do not under any circumstances recommend that you use mandrake for medicinal purposes of any kind, as all parts of the plant are highly toxic. Mandrake should be grown only for magical or religious use, and certainly not in an area where children or pets could have access to it and possibly ingest it.

Herbs on the Web

~ By Roslyn Reid ~

I will begin by assuming that anyone reading this article is somewhat conversant with the internet, and I won't bother explaining basic concepts. If you are not familiar with the internet and would like to be, try consulting "Internet for Dummies," or just get online and fool around—it's all pretty easy to learn.

Meanwhile, I'll continue. As with many subjects, the internet has numerous websites devoted to gardening. But as with any other data gathered from the internet, the slogan here should be "Surfer Beware." Much useful information is available if one is careful to evaluate the source, but one should never assume all information is good just because it was found on a website— no matter how impressive that site looks. For instance, commercial sites have good tips, but only if you keep in mind that the real purpose of such sites

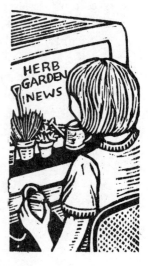

is to sell you something. The information you obtain on any such site is likely to steer you toward products or services sold by a particular company. For this reason, nonprofit, government, or educational websites can be better sources of information. Commercial websites usually are distinguished by the ".com" extension in their addresses; but be aware that their URLs may also end in ".net," or some other suffix. Nonprofits generally use the extension ".org;" federal sites use ".gov;" and colleges and other institutes of learning use the extension ".edu."

When using a global tool like the internet for an activity as regional as gardening, you need to determine if any information gathered is applicable to your location. Check for a two-letter country codes at the end of the address, or whether a site is state-based—such as "www.state.nj.us." Then, use your best judgment to determine whether the data on the page is pertinent to your area. Keep in mind that the ubiquity of the internet can be helpful to gardeners—there are no seasons on the internet, after all, and the information is always avaiable so that even in the winter you can learn about your garden.

Generally, the following criteria for evaluating websites were used for this article:

Speed—This is probably the biggest complaint about the World Wide Web—it can be slow. Many webmasters think a black background is a cool way to show off their spiffy graphics. My experience is that this—as well as all those spiffy graphics—slows the download and makes printing out the page difficult. In many instances, elaborate graphics or photos are better when reduced to small clickable thumbnails. I also believe some "features" such as java tickers or music are better left out—most of the time they seem to be included just to demonstrate that the web page designer is oh so clever. Advertising banners also slow a page down, although they are usually necessary evils to pay the bills. There are a lot of ads out there now, and many of are them irrelevant.

Ease of Navigation—Can you find information easily without having to browse through many confusing or unnecessary pages? Many sites make you click through lots of superfluous pages before you find the information you are seeking. Watch sites for a search feature or site map, so you can quickly locate what you need.

Quality of Information—Is the information useful, or just a sales pitch? Is the data in-depth or sketchy? Are the assertions based on fact, or just speculation? And who is the target audience—landscape architects? Home gardeners? Folklore enthusiasts? Make sure you don't waste your time searching through data that is too far above or below your level of knowledge.

Special Features—Extra features on a website are only useful when they add to your search—chat rooms? Ask-an-expert section? E-mail for questions you may have? Links to similar sites? References or bibliography? Their usefulness depends on your needs.

General Sites

Now on to our review of some popular herb-related websites. These have been broken down into four categories: general (with the subcategories of commercial and non-commercial), specialty, tours, and unusual. Keep in mind that the internet is in a constant state of change—some of these websites may disappear by the time this article is published, and hundreds added.

Commercial General Sites

Note: a "privacy policy" is a disclosure commercial sites should make about how they will use any information you supply them with. The existence of this policy, or its lack, will be noted for each commercial site mentioned below.

BetterLawns.com (www.betterlawns.com)—This is the website of Tom MacCubbin, host of a popular Florida radio show on gardening. The site includes a real audio feature for listening to shows, a search feature, a gardening Q&A, and links—mostly to universities.

Burpee (www.burpee.com)—A privacy policy is posted in the "customer service" section. This is a lush site with a garden tour, recipes, and a photo contest. Weekly regional gardening reports cover all areas in the U.S. There is also a Q&A database. Besides seeds, Burpee also sells herbs in plant form; but there is no search feature.

Garden.com (www.garden.com)—A privacy policy is posted. Many graphics slow down the loading of this large site, primarily intended for shopping. There is also lot of non product-related information—such as garden planning help, an online magazine, a Q&A, a question submission form, chat rooms, and a search feature.

Gardener's Supply Company (www.gardeners.com)—The privacy policy is posted. This company sells equipment, seeds, medical items, and crafts. With the exception of the articles in the "Gardener's News" section, most of the gardening information here is product-related. There is a search form and an online newsletter.

Garden Net (www.gardennet.com)—This is a good starting point—a huge site with links to practically everything that also loads quickly due to minimal graphics. There is a chat room, a form to request catalogs from many companies, links, and a list of public gardens. Local data and ideas on where to obtain further information are available.

Gardens Alive! (www.gardens-alive.com)—The privacy policy is posted. This site sells organic gardening products such as fertilizers, but the shopping section loads very slowly. Also included: a list of county extension agents for across the U.S., gardening tips, and a search feature. There are excellent pictures of garden pests and diseases.

GardenWeb (www.gardenweb.com)—This site has lots of general information. It loads quickly due to minimal graphics and no ads, and has links to every conceivable gardening subject. There is no site search feature, but it does have a "quick index." Material on herbs can be found in the plant dictionary, the forums, and the garden directory. There is also a "mystery plant" contest.

Horticultural Web (www.horticulture.com)—This site is meant for professionals, but advanced amateurs can make use of it. Information is drawn heavily from university sources. There are lots of links, but they are hard to find. There is also a multi-vendor shopping section, so the privacy policy for each vendor must be checked. The site itself does not have a posted policy.

I Can Garden (www.icangarden.com)—This Canadian site includes articles and links on everything you can imagine—including black tomatoes! There is a search feature, an international events calendar, and articles on herbs.

Jerry Baker's Gardening for Life (www.jerrybaker.com)—The privacy policy is posted. Altthough this is a shopping site, you can find Jerry's famous free information on low-cost gardening solutions. His extensive appearance schedule is also posted. The site is updated weekly and includes a question submission form, a gardening Q&A, gardening tips, an online newsletter, a garden contest, and search feature. You can also find information on Jerry's gardening scholarships,but there are no links.

Johnny's Selected Seeds (www.johnnyseeds.com)—No privacy policy is posted. Limited graphics make this site load quickly. Lots of herb seeds are available, including rarities such as thistle and organic seeds. There are gardening tips, links to other sites, and even a tour of the company facilities! Johnny's offers internet specials on its seeds and plant products. This site is a member of the

Herb Web Ring, which enables you to jump to other herb sites by clicking on the links at the bottom of the page.

Mellinger's (www.mellingers.com)—No privacy policy is posted. This company sells plants and gardening products, and their site loads fairly fast. They carry cooking herbs, and handle a good selection of unusual plants. There are notable online specials, a search feature, and e-mail. There is limited information on gardening.

Seedman.com (www.seedman.com)—The privacy policy is posted. This site has an interesting selection of seeds— including rose, banana, tobacco, and loofah—offered by subject area, such as tea or cooking. Certain herbs, such as stevia, have their own pages. Bulk seeds are available.

The Trellis (www.wormsway.com/trellis.html)—Here you will find more than 150 gardening links, but there is no search feature. There is information on herbariums.

Walt Nicke's Garden Talk (www.gardentalk.com)—No privacy policy posted. Sells gardening equipment but not plants. The site loads quickly, but you can only order a limited number of items, leave comments, or read the "Garden Stories" page on this site. More is promised.

Non-Commercial General Sites

United States Department of Agriculture (www.usda.gov)— This site has minimal graphics and loads quickly. The search function yields articles on growing and using herbs.

Urban Agriculture Notes (www.cityfarmer.org)—This is a huge Canadian site with lots of information. Fortunately, there is a search feature. The site also includes pictures, inks, garden tours, and even video.

Specialty Sites

Botanical.com (www.botanical.com)—This is an excellent site with full hypertext version of Mrs. Grieve's *A*

Modern Herbal. There are lots of links, and various articles on alternative medicine and other uses of herbs, as well as conversion tables for cooking.

Flowerweb Flowerbase (www.flowerbase.com)—Enter a plant name here, and the site will bring up its picture and some information for you. However, the pictures of flowering herbs are quite unclear and obscured by text.

Heirloom Seeds (www.heirloomseeds.com)—This is a very nice site from a Pennsylvania company that sells "old-time" non-hybrid seeds. One of their offerings is a medicinal herb package. There is a question submission form, garden tip contest, newsletter, and local information, but they have an odd ordering system.

Herbal Encyclopedia (www.wic.net/waltzark/herbenc.htm)—This is one instance where a picture makes an annoying background. Nevertheless, there is lots of information on herbs here, divided into three sections: medicinal, religious, and growing. There is no search feature, but there is an alphabetical list of herbs, and links to various articles.

Traditional Gardening (www.traditionalgardening.com)—This site has selected online articles devoted to period gardening. There is a search feature, a question submission form, and links to suppliers. Herbal information can be found in the "Archives" link, usually in the "From the Kitchen Garden" column. There is an "Herb Supplier" search category.

Tours

Brooklyn Botanic Garden (www.bbg.org)—This is an excellent virtual garden tour. There is a search feature, bibliography, links, and a shop. Oddly enough, no privacy policy is posted. Special attention is paid to urban plants. Some of the most comprehensive information available concerning online shopping and other internet-related topics can be found on this site.

The Telegarden (www.usc.edu/dept/garden)—This site concerns robot education, and students use robots to take a virtual garden tour. The robot is controlled by the user over the internet. The idea of gardening by robot is so unique and interesting, I thought it worth a mention.

Unusual Sites

Gothic Gardening (www.gothic.net/~malice)—Some sites with black backgrounds are still worth it, and this is one of them. It has advice on growing poison nightshade, information on the ancient beliefs about mandrake root and great links to herbal lore, among other things.

Ketzel Levine's Talking Plants (talkingplants.com)—This is the website of a popular PBS show. It's also a hoot. Included are a rather long survey, as well as a new interview every week. In the interview are links to informational sites on the plants mentioned—some of which are herbs. Unfortunately, the excellent and informative "Plant Profiles" section is mostly dedicated to flowers. The shopping section, with its offbeat bug sculptures for the garden, is not to be missed! No privacy policy is posted.

To Conclude

Of necessity, this article has provided only a very brief tour of some of the thousands of herb-related sites available on the internet. I hope readers will find these reviews a good starting point. Once you become comfortable finding your way around, you will be able to locate many more interesting sites and share them with your fellow herbalists and gardeners.

Dragon Plants

☙ By Eileen Holland ❧

Witches use the four ele-ments—earth, air, fire and water—in magical prac-tice. Dragons can represent each one. For instance:

Air: Winged dragons that fly

Fire: Fire-breathing dragons

Water: Sea serpent dragons

Earth: Treasure-guarding dragons who live in caves (such as Tolkien's Smaug).

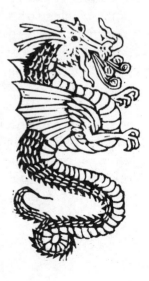

Dragons are considered negative in Celtic lore but are positive in Eastern traditions—as portents of luck, pros-perity, fertility, and enlightenment. If you have experienced the joyous dragon dance on Chinese New Year, you have some understanding of this belief.

You may not believe in dragons but you can work with the idea of them if you like. The Chinese discipline of feng-shui, for example, utilizes the world dragon's breath and our position on its back. Witches and other magical people use dragons as paths to the elements. Plants can be a gateway for working with dragon-energies. Dragon's blood and bistort, also called dragonwort, are excellent for this. Either one can be used to activate this prayer.

Dragon Blessing

May dragons bring me wealth
and guard my treasures
May they banish darkness and enlighten me
May female dragons grant me inner power
May the Dragon Queen neutralize my enemies
May Dragon Spirits give me power over Elementals
May weather dragons bring rain at my request
May Ti'amat effect the changes I command
May Ishtar grant me Dragon Power
May Ishtar grant me Dragon Power

Dragon's Blood

You'll find lots of things called dragon's blood for sale, but true dragon's blood is only produced by plants of the Croton, Daemonorops and Dracena families. It is used in magic for: inner power, strength, will power, manifesting changes, love spells, exorcism, binding spells, protection, self-defense, energy, dragon magic, potency, empowering amulets, talismans, or spells, male sex magic, yang energy, consecrating tools, courage, animal magic, purification, cleansing, luck, and money spells.

True Dragon's blood corresponds to the planet Mars, the element Fire, and the sign Aries. Dragon's blood has male energy and is a charm against impotence. It can be used in charms and spells, sprinkled around the home, or added to a liquid for floor washes. Burned as incense, dragon's blood resin banishes evil, dispels negativity and wins lovers back, and it strengthens the virtues of other kinds of incense. Washing with dragon's blood soap or adding dragon's blood oil to the bath purifies it.

Plants that provide Dracon's Blood

Dragon Tree (Dracena draco)—Dragon trees, which resemble palms, are one of the oldest plants in existence. They grow to gigantic size in their natural habitat of the Canary Islands and the East Indies, reaching 70 feet tall and 45 feet around. Their trunks and lower branches are bare. A rosette of thick, stiff, palmate leaves grows from the top. These fleshy leaves that are sometimes outlined in red, grow to two feet long. Dragon trees bloom with greenish white flowers that look like clusters of lilies. The fruit is an orange berry. Dark red dragon's blood seeps from cracks in the trunks of the trees. When dried it burns with a bright flame. Dragon trees live long lives—one tree in Tenerife was reputed to be over 6000 years old. Dragon trees are propagated by seed, dislike isolation and excessive humidity. They can be grown as houseplants.

Uses—Dragon's blood resin was employed to color varnishes, especially those used by Italian violin makers. It was also once used in photoengraving. The Guanche people of the Canary Islands held dragon trees sacred, and used the resin in embalming.

Socotrine Dragon's Blood, Guadeloupe Dragon's Blood (Dracena cinnabari)—An African tree, native to the island of Socotra, east of Somalia, and the East Indies and South America. It produces small, irregular lumps of dragon's blood resin called Socotrine Dragon's Blood or Zanzibar Drop. This tree was once classified as Pterocarpus Draco.

Chinese Dragon's Blood (Dracena terminalis)—Asian tree that yields dragon's blood resin. The syrup of its roots induces sweating, treats dysentery, and diarrhea, and sugar made from the roots can be fermented to produce an alcoholic drink. The resin provides a red varnish.

Dragon's Blood Palm, Tear Dragon's Blood, Draconis Resina, Sanguis Draconis, Calamus Gum, Calamus Draco (Daemonorops draco)—The rattan palm tree, native to Malaysia and Indonesia, has pointed berries providing dragon's blood resin. It has spiny leaves and bark, blooms with flowers along its branches.

The resin is harvested by steaming the berries or by rubbing their coatings off. Tear Dragon's Blood is a beaded 'necklace' formed of berry coats. The resin is also sold powdered, in lumps, or molded into sticks. The resin is very brittle and breaks easily. Fresh resin is painted on wounds to stop bleeding, protect against infection, and promote healing. An astringent, it can be used internally for irregular menstruation, traumatic injuries, and to stop bleeding after childbirth or miscarriage. The tree provides rattan for wickerwork. The resin can be used to color varnish, lacquers and other products.

Dragon's Blood Palm (Daemonorops didynophyllys, Daemonorops micranthus, Daemonorops propingaus)—Malaysian palm trees whose immature fruits provide dragon's blood resin.

Blood of the Dragon, Drago, Sangre de Grado, Sangre de Drago (Croton lechleri)—Tall tree of tropical South America, especially the Amazon rainforest, with green, heart-shaped leaves. Its pale, mottled bark leaks dragon's blood latex when cut. It blooms with long stalks of greenish white flowers. The bark and resin are antibacterial, antiseptic, anti-inflammatory, and anti-viral. Both are used in folk medicine for digestive ulcers, as a vaginal douche, for wounds and skin diseases. Dragon's blood latex is painted on wounds to disinfect them, stop bleeding, and promote healing. An alkaloid called taspine is the active ingredient. The antiviral drugs Provir and Virend are made from this tree.

Other varieties providing dragon's blood include: Croton salutaris, Croton planostigma, Croton draconoides, Croton erythrochilus, Croton salutaris, Croton hibiscifolius, Croton sanguifolius.

Bistort

From the Latin for "twice twisted," referring to the herb's often S-shaped roots, Bistort meant is an herb of Saturn and the Sun; its quality is cold and dry. The root is used magically for: psychic work, psychic power, dragon magic, serpent power, divination, trance work, fertility. Bistort root is a charm against heartbreak and eye problems. It is said to have a calming effect when carried near the heart, and to make men perform sexually. Touching the root gives you the all virtues of your sign or planet. Both leaves and roots are a charm against poison.

Bistort, Bistort Root, Great Bistort, Dragon's Wort, Serpentary, Snakeweed, Snake Root, Adderwort, Osterick, Passions, Oderwort, Easter Mangiant, Twice Writhen, Serpentaria, Columbrina, Dracunculus, Patience Dock (Polygon um bistorta)—Bistort is a perennial Eurasian herb that grows to twenty inches. Its large oval leaves are bluish green with ashy undersides. The plant favors colder climates, growing in moist, shady places—woods, damp meadows, near waterways. Bistort blooms spring to autumn, with dense cylindrical spikes of small pinkish or white flowers on long slender stems. The twisted rootstock is about two inches long, with a blackish or dark purple exterior and reddish brown flesh. Small shiny brown seeds are encased in three-sided fruits. Gather and dry the root early in the spring. Gather the leaves in spring or fall; harvest seeds when they ripen. Bistort is a medicinally useful herb whose root contains the most active principle. It is full of tannin, a strong astringent. It is used to treat nosebleeds, nasal infections, cystitis, cholera, colitis, diarrhea, dysentery, hemorrhoids, internal and heavy menstrual bleeding. Bistort can be made into a gargle for sore throat, gum diseases, mouth ulcers and loose teeth; into an ointment for anal fissures or a douche for vaginal discharges. Nicholas Culpepper, the 17th century English astrological botanist, recommended distilled water of leaves for bites, stings, running sores and skin ulcers. The root was also used in tanning leather.

American Bistort (Polygonum bistortoides)—This is an alpine and sub-alpine Eurasian herb with long, narrow leaves. It grows to one foot or more, and blooms with flowers on leafed stalks. The long root is black and crinkled. American Bistort grows wild beside streams in northwestern North America.

Other Dragon Plants

Dracena, which means female dragon. Dracena are

woody-stemmed plants of the tropical eastern hemisphere. They have orange or yellow roots, a crown of leathery leaves, and bloom with clusters of small white flowers. They like moist roots and a warm climate, are propagated by cuttings or stem sections. There are many varieties of dracena, most of which can be grown indoors as houseplants.

Dragon Queen, Queen of Dracenas (Dracena goldioana)—African plant with thin canes that grows to ten feet. It has a rosette of glossy, leathery leaves that are deep green with pale green markings. Dragon Queen blooms at night with fragrant white flowers. It needs porous soil and a humid climate.

Madagascar Dragon Tree (Dracena marginata)—Branching, tree-like plant with a rosette of fleshy leaves atop slender, twisting, cane-like trunks. It grows slowly, reaching twelve feet in height. The deep olive green leaves have red edges.

Arabic: om Beit, or Mother of the Bouse (Dracena ombet)—Small tree-like plant with sword-shaped leaves. The stem and branches are forked. It blooms with panicles of delicate pink flowers. The fruit is a round berry.

Dragon Lily (Dracena fragrans)—A rare plant that grows in the mountains near Sudan. It is often cultivated as a houseplant.

Gold Dust Dracena (Dracena goddsefiana)—A shrubby plant with whorls of thin, leathery, deep green leaves that are glossy and have yellow spots. It blooms with greenish yellow flowers. The fruit is a red berry.

Ribbon Plant (Dracena sanderiana)—A small plant with a rosette of thin, deep green leaves.

Traditional Celtic Herbalism

By Ellen Evert Hopman

Restoring Airmid's Cloak

The foundation myth of the Celtic herbalist's art is the story of Diancecht and his children Airmid and Miach. Diancecht, a Celtic God of medicine, became jealous when his son Miach's reputation began to eclipse his own. In a fit of rage Diancecht hit his son on the head with a sword but Miach easily healed himself. Diancecht attacked a second time, cutting to the bone, but Miach cured himself again. Finally, Diancecht clove his son's head in two, and this time killed him.

Diancecht buried his son and three hundred and sixty five healing herbs sprang from Miach's body, possibly a reference to a now-lost astronomical plant classification system. Airmid, Miach's sister, harvested the herbs and arranged them on her cloak in the shape of a human being to show where they were useful to the human body.

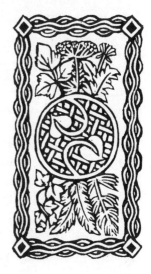

Ever jealous, Diancecht kicked the cloak and scattered the herbs, thus confusing their meanings. If not for his actions, according to the ancients, we would know the cure for every illness and so be immortal. Every herbalist working with herbs today is engaged in the work of restoring Airmid's cloak—the knowledge that was once a part of every child's basic education. Another mystery encoded in this story is that as Miach, the young God, dwells under the earth, so every healing plant that springs from the soil is a living part of his body. When an herbalist gathers plants she is dismembering the god. When she administers them to the sick she is ritually reuniting the lost pieces of the god and bringing the world back into wholeness.

To understand which herbs might have formed the figure on Airmid's cloak we can begin by looking at the pollen record from one of the most important archaeological sites of ancient Ireland— Newgrange, near Slane, in County Meath. Built in approximately 3,500 b.c. on the Boyne river, the funerary complex of Newgrange was surrounded by the villages and settlements of the people who constructed it. The pollen taken from the excavation has left a record of which plants were native to the area. As the Celts moved into Ireland they would have learned the uses of these herbs from indigenous healers. The pollen record shows that nettles, mint, Saint John's wort, hazel, dock, wormwood, ivy, linden, horsetail, bedstraw, birch, willow, and oak were among the plants available to local herbalists.

Herbs of the Ancient Celts

Nettles (Urtica spp.)—Nettles was an important iron-rich food for the ancients, used as a pot herb and in soups and stews, or as a tea antihistamine and antinflamatory for allergies and rheumatism.

Mints (Mentha spp.)—Mint tea was used as a beverage and as a cure for diarrhea. Mixed with elder flowers and yarrow blossoms it made a classic remedy for fever and flu. Mint was useful in colic and indigestion and as an emmenagogue. A mint wash was soothing to burns and sunburn.

Saint John's wort (Hypericum perforatum)—With its yellow star-like flowers that bleed red when crushed, Saint John's wort was considered an herb of the Sun gods Belenos and Belisama, and a wound wort. The flowers were used in salves for burns and skin irritations and taken as a tea for melancholy. In modern times too it is becoming widely known as an antidepressant, but it should be avoided by persons already on synthetic medications that are MAO inhibitors. Prolonged use will cause photophobia, an increased sensitivity to sunlight. Try using kava kava and damiana in the bright summer months. The Welsh called it "The Herb of the Blessed" because it was thought to be the ideal combination of fire and water—the basic elements out of which the universe was created. When fire and water, light and dark were present in equal measure there was a great potential for transformative magic and healing. The ancients picked this herb at Midsummer (June 21) and bathed it in the smoke of a ritual fire. Later it was hung in the home and barn to keep madness and all evil at bay. It was also sewn into power bundles to be worn as a protective charm.

In Breton tradition a power bundle contained nine grains of salt and the leaves of nine plants. Each plant was associated with a different god or goddess and a different part of the body—vervain for the head, perhaps because it cured colds and sore throats; Saint John's wort for the blood, because it bleeds when crushed; greater celandine and eyebright for the eyes; chamomile for the breasts; pennyroyal for the lungs; lemon balm for the heart; and hepatica for the liver. Mugwort or yarrow were associated with the waist because of their effects on the female reproductive tract and the small intestines, and male fern with the bowels because of its anti parasitic effects. Ivy, scarlet pimpernel, fumitory, white clover, field daisy and cinquefoil were also used. The bag contained a coin and was sewn shut with a flaxen thread. In Celtic folk tradition a gold coin signified the powers of the sun and a silver coin the powers of the moon.

Hazel Tree (Corylus avellana)—This tree was one of the "nine sacred woods" of Celtic ritual. The major Celtic holidays (Samhain/Halloween, Imbolc/Candlemas, Beltaine/May Day, Lughnasad/First Fruits) were all known as Fire Festivals and were characterized by the building of bonfires on hilltops. Each ritual fire was kindled by a fire drill made of oak.

Three or nine sacred woods were used as fuel in these fires. The *Carmina Gadelica* (a collection of prayers and incantations from the Highlands and Islands of Scotland by Alexander Carmichael) lists them as; "Willow of the streams, hazel of the rocks, alder of the marshes, birch of the waterfalls, rowan of the shade, the yew of resilience, elm of the brae, oak of the sun". The ninth tree may have been holly, ash, or pine.

Hazel was especially associated with sacred springs and wells. For the ancient Celts, water was the entrance to the Otherworld, and offerings could be made to the ancestors and the Gods by placing hazel nuts or other offerings into lakes and wells. In the early Irish Dindsenchas we read of Connla's Well, located near Tipperary. The Nine Hazels of Poetry hung over it, dropping their flowers (beauty) and fruit (wisdom) into the waters. Sacred salmon living in the well swallowed the nuts as they fell, developing one bright spot for every nut they consumed. The nuts were said to give birth to every science and art.

Hazel was one of the Seven Chieftain Trees of Ireland, the cutting of which was punishable by the fine of one cow. The ancient Brehon Laws list the seven trees as: oak, for its beauty and size and because its acorns are food for pigs; hazel for its wattles and nuts; apple for its bark which was used in tanning; yew for its timber used for bows, breastplates, and household implements; holly because its wood made the shafts of chariots; ash because its wood made weapons and the royal throne; and pine for flooring and casks.

Hazel was a traditional wood for dowsing wands used to divine water sources. The nuts were eaten before divination and Druids were said to carry them on their person. Diancecht, the

God of healing, invented a porridge for the sick that was reputed to cure colds, sore throats and worms. According to legend it consisted of hazel buds, dandelions, chickweed, sorrel, and oatmeal. It was taken mornings and evenings.

Dandelions were sacred to the Goddess Brighid because they had a milky sap. Her festival, Imbolc (Candlemas), marked the onset of the lactation of the ewes. Often worshiped at holy wells, Brighid was a Goddess of healing.

Yellowdock (Rumex crispus)—"Dock" was an excellent blood tonic. Spring gathered, it was cleansing to the blood and fall gathered it added iron. The flesh of the root was an ideal tonic laxative and iron supplement for pregnancy. It also benefited liver disorders, rheumatism, hemorrhoids and anemia. The outer peel of the root and the seeds benefited diarrhea.

Wormwood (Artemisia absynthum)—Wormwood leaves and flowers were made into a light tea for digestive upsets. The tea also helped relieve labor pains and expelled worms. Externally the herb was used to poultice bruises, sprains and arthritis. (Use this herb with caution as prolonged use can lead to nerve damage). Wormwood has traditionally been thought of as a psychic aid. It was burned in a graveyard to summon the spirits of the ancestors. The herb was hung and strewn about the house as an insect repellent.

Ivy (Hedera helix)—Ivy twigs were simmered into salves for burns. The leaves made a douche for vaginal infections. Externally it was used to poultice damaged nerves, sinews, ulcers, enlarged glands, boils, and abscesses. Ivy's ability to remain green in the winter was regarded as magical. Ivy hoops and wreaths were woven and placed in and among the milk containers. Wreaths of ivy, rowan (mountain ash), and woodbine were hung over the entrance to barns and cattle pens as a protection for the beasts. The bruised plant was strewn and hung to discourage lice and other vermin.

Linden Tree (Lime Tree) (Tilia europea)—Linden flowers made a calming and relaxing brew. The wood of the tree was used for matting, baskets, fishnets, shoes, ropes, and bridles. The root bark was soothing for burns and the flowers eased nervous vomiting, heart palpitations, spasms, headaches, cough,s and pains. The buds were edible as a food. Linden flower honey had relaxing properties.

Horsetail (Equisetum spp.)—Spring-gathered horsetail was a great source of nourishment for skin, hair, bones, teeth, bladder, kidney, and prostate. It made a soothing wash for conjunctivitis and was useful as a tea for fevers. The ash of the plant was used as an abrasive "toothpaste."

Bedstraw (Galium aparine)—Bedstraw could be eaten fresh or taken as a tea for eczema, psoriasis, and kidney disorders. Externally it made a poultice for tumors and inflammations.

Birch Tree (Betula spp.)—The Gaelic word for birch, "beith," is related to the word "bith," which means enduring or constant, and to the word "bithe," or womanly. Birch was traditionally regarded as a feminine tree, associated with goddesses. Birch wood was used to make tool handles, brooms and barrels. The twigs were used for thatching. Birch leaf tea was mildly laxative, cleared sediments from the kidney and bladder, and relieved rheumatism and mouth sores. A strong brew of the twigs, leaves and bark could be used as a wash for eczema, psoriasis, and other moist skin eruptions. When using leaves from deciduous trees they must be picked before the Summer Solstice, June 21. Leaves picked after that date will have strong concentrations of natural insecticides that can prove irritating to human tissue.

Willow Tree (Salix spp.)—"Sally" from the Gaelic "Saille," was used to make baskets, fencing, sieves for winnowing grain, frames for coracles (leather boats) and for roof thatching. The modern drug "aspirin" is actually a synthetic form of willow bark. All willow contain the glycoside salicin which is the "active ingredient" in aspirin. Willow bark tea was used to lower fevers, soothe muscle pains and inflammations, and relieve rheumatic complaints. It made a gargle for sore throats and an external wash for wounds, burns, and sores. The sap of the flowering tree was drunk or used as a wash for the eyes.

Oak Tree (Quercus spp.)—The oak tree was one of the most important building materials for shelters and homes. A dense firewood, it was also vital for giving heat. Its acorns were an important source of carbohydrates for humans, pigs, and game. Oak wood was used to fashion spears, bows, oars, and boats. The bark and leaf were boiled into an astringent brew to tan hides and fish nets. The same brew made a powerful wound wash that pulled the edges of a wound together. White oak bark tea was taken internally for coughs, colds and to clear phlegm from the system. The oak tree had many sacred associations for the Celts. Known to attract lightening, it was sacred to sky gods associated with thunder. The dead were buried in oak coffins or in the hollowed out trunk of ancient oaks. Among the Gaulish Celts, mistletoe found growing on oak was especially venerated. According to Pliny, two white oxen were sacrificed when the "all heal" was found. It was ritually cut on the "sixth day of the moon" by a Druid dressed in white, using a "golden sickle" (which must have been bronze as gold is too soft). The plant was caught by another Druid waiting below with a cloth to keep it from touching the ground. Tradition states that carrying acorns on your person or keeping them in the house will bring good luck.

Making Herbal Salves

Modern herbalists make healing salves for burns and skin irritations, diaper rash, and eczema out of bees wax and olive oil. Herbs such as comfrey, plantain, calendula, elecampagne root, and lavender are placed in a non aluminum pot, covered with good-quality olive oil, and simmered for twenty minutes using a tight lid. A separate pot filled with bees wax is brought to a simmer and when both liquids are the same temperature three tablespoons of beeswax are added for every cup of olive oil used. The mixture is strained into jars and stored away from light.

The ancient Celts probably used butter or lard as the foundation of their healing salves. When I was in Ireland researching one of my books I was privileged to meet Johnny Mulherne in Straduffy Cross, Kiltyclogher. Johnnie was widely regarded as the most prominent traditional healer of his locality. His specialty was shingles, a painful nerve inflammation. His reputation was such that even a bishop had once come to him for a cure.

At the time he gave me this formula, Johnny was in his nineties and healthy enough to take me on an herb walk to show me the plants he used. His eyes were still sharp and his memory clear. He recommended boiling the herbs in butter for eighteen hours, praying over the pot, and also praying over the lesions of the one who was sick.

Traditional Irish Shingles Remedy

Ingredients: Scutch Grass (Agropyron repens)—also known as Witch Grass, Couch Grass, Cutch, Dog Grass, Durfa Grass, Quack Grass, Quick Grass, and Triticum.

Shamrock (Oxalis acetosella)—also known as Common sorrel, Cuckoo bread, Green sauce, Mountain sorrel, Sour trefoil, Stubwort, White sorrel.

Yellow dock (Rumex crispus)—also known as Curled dock, Garden patience, Narrow dock, Sour dock, Rumex.

Male fern (Dryopteris Felix-mas, or Aspidium Filix-mas)—also known as Aspidium, Bear's paw root, Knotty brake, Sweet brake.

Primrose (Primula officinalis)—also known as Butter rose, English cowslip.

Boot tree, or elder, bark (Sambucus nigra)—also known as Black elder, European elder, Boor tree, Country elder, Bounty, Ellan wood, Elihorn, German elder. American Elder (Sambucus canadensis) can be used as a substitute.

Hound's Tongue (Cynoglossum officinale)—also known as Dog-bur, Dog's tongue, Gypsy flower, sheep lice, wool mat.

Pennyroyal (Hedeoma puiegioides)—also known as American pennyroyal, Mock pennyroyal, Mosquito plant, Squaw balm, Squaw mint, Tick weed.

Strawberry—Use the whole plant except for the root.

Simmer the herbs in butter, strain through a cheese cloth and store in glass jars in a cool, dark place.

The Quarters and Signs of the Moon and Moon Tables

The Quarters and Signs of the Moon

*E*veryone has seen the Moon wax and wane through a period of approximately twenty-nine and-a-half days. This circuit from New Moon to Full Moon and back again is called the lunation cycle. The cycle is divided into parts, called quarters or phases. There are several methods by which this can be done, and the system used in the *Herbal Almanac* may not correspond to those used in other almanacs.

The Quarters

First Quarter

The first quarter begins at the New Moon, when the Sun and Moon are in the same place, or conjunct. (This means that the Sun and Moon are in the same degree of the same sign.) The Moon is not visible at first, since it rises at the same time as the Sun. The New Moon is the time of new beginnings, beginnings of projects that favor growth, externalization of activities, and the growth of ideas. The first quarter is the time of germination, emergence, beginnings, and outwardly directed activity.

Second Quarter

The second quarter begins halfway between the New Moon and the Full Moon, when the Sun and Moon are at right angles, or a 90 degree square to each other. This half Moon rises around noon and sets around midnight, so it can be seen in the western sky during the first half of the night. The second quarter is the time of growth and articulation of things that already exist.

Third Quarter

The third quarter begins at the Full Moon, when the Sun and Moon are opposite one another and the full light of the Sun can shine on the full sphere of the Moon. The round Moon can be seen rising in the east at sunset, and then rising a little later each evening. The Full Moon stands for illumination, fulfillment, culmination, completion, drawing inward, unrest, emotional expressions, and hasty actions leading to failure. The third quarter is a time of maturity, fruition, and the assumption of the full form of expression.

Fourth Quarter

The fourth quarter begins about halfway between the Full Moon and New Moon, when the Sun and Moon are again at 90 degrees, or square. This decreasing Moon rises at midnight, and can be seen in the east during the last half of the night, reaching the overhead position just about as the Sun rises. The fourth quarter is a time of disintegration, drawing back for reorganization and reflection.

The Signs

Moon in Aries

Moon in Aries is good for starting things, but lacking in staying power. Things occur rapidly, but also quickly pass.

Moon in Taurus

With Moon in Taurus, things begun during this sign last the longest and tend to increase in value. Things begun now become habitual and hard to alter.

Moon in Gemini

Moon in Gemini is an inconsistent position for the Moon, characterized by a lot of talk. Things begun now are easily changed by outside influences.

Moon in Cancer

Moon in Cancer stimulates emotional rapport between people. It pinpoints need, and supports growth and nurturance.

Moon in Leo

Moon in Leo accents showmanship, being seen, drama, recreation, and happy pursuits. It may be concerned with praise and subject to flattery.

Moon in Virgo

Moon in Virgo favors accomplishment of details and commands from higher up while discouraging independent thinking.

Moon in Libra

Moon in Libra increases self-awareness. It favors self-examination and interaction with others, but discourages spontaneous initiative.

Moon in Scorpio

Moon in Scorpio increases awareness of psychic power. It precipitates psychic crises and ends connections thoroughly.

Moon in Sagittarius

Moon in Sagittarius encourages expansionary flights of imagination and confidence in the flow of life.

Moon in Capricorn

Moon in Capricorn increases awareness of the need for structure, discipline, and organization. Institutional activities are favored.

Moon in Aquarius

Moon in Aquarius favors activities that are unique and individualistic, concern for humanitarian needs, society as a whole, and improvements that can be made.

Moon in Pisces

During Moon in Pisces, energy withdraws from the surface of life, hibernates within, secretly reorganizing and realigning.

January Moon Table

Date	Sign	Element	Nature	Phase
1 Mon. 5:14 pm	Aries	Fire	Barren	1st
2 Tue.	Aries	Fire	Barren	2nd 5:31 pm
3 Wed.	Aries	Fire	Barren	2nd
4 Thu. 1:57 am	Taurus	Earth	Semi-fruit	2nd
5 Fri.	Taurus	Earth	Semi-fruit	2nd
6 Sat. 6:44 am	Gemini	Air	Barren	2nd
7 Sun.	Gemini	Air	Barren	2nd
8 Mon. 8:09 am	Cancer	Water	Fruitful	2nd
9 Tue.	Cancer	Water	Fruitful	3rd 3:24 pm
10 Wed. 7:44 am	Leo	Fire	Barren	3rd
11 Thu.	Leo	Fire	Barren	3rd
12 Fri. 7:26 am	Virgo	Earth	Barren	3rd
13 Sat.	Virgo	Earth	Barren	3rd
14 Sun. 9:05 am	Libra	Air	Semi-fruit	3rd
15 Mon.	Libra	Air	Semi-fruit	3rd
16 Tue. 2:02 pm	Scorpio	Water	Fruitful	4th 7:35 am
17 Wed.	Scorpio	Water	Fruitful	4th
18 Thu. 10:35 pm	Sagittarius	Fire	Barren	4th
19 Fri.	Sagittarius	Fire	Barren	4th
20 Sat.	Sagittarius	Fire	Barren	4th
21 Sun. 9:57 am	Capricorn	Earth	Semi-fruit	4th
22 Mon.	Capricorn	Earth	Semi-fruit	4th
23 Tue. 10:43 pm	Aquarius	Air	Barren	4th
24 Wed.	Aquarius	Air	Barren	1st 8:07 am
25 Thu.	Aquarius	Air	Barren	1st
26 Fri. 11:39 am	Pisces	Water	Fruitful	1st
27 Sat.	Pisces	Water	Fruitful	1st
28 Sun. 11:35 pm	Aries	Fire	Barren	1st
29 Mon.	Aries	Fire	Barren	1st
30 Tue.	Aries	Fire	Barren	1st
31 Wed. 9:21 am	Taurus	Earth	Semi-fruit	1st

February Moon Table

Date	Sign	Element	Nature	Phase
1 Thu.	Taurus	Earth	Semi-fruit	2nd 9:02 am
2 Fri. 3:56 pm	Gemini	Air	Barren	2nd
3 Sat.	Gemini	Air	Barren	2nd
4 Sun. 7:00 pm	Cancer	Water	Fruitful	2nd
5 Mon.	Cancer	Water	Fruitful	2nd
6 Tue. 7:21 pm	Leo	Fire	Barren	2nd
7 Wed.	Leo	Fire	Barren	2nd
8 Thu. 6:35 pm	Virgo	Earth	Barren	3rd 2:12 am
9 Fri.	Virgo	Earth	Barren	3rd
10 Sat. 6:46 pm	Libra	Air	Semi-fruit	3rd
11 Sun.	Libra	Air	Semi-fruit	3rd
12 Mon. 9:51 pm	Scorpio	Water	Fruitful	3rd
13 Tue.	Scorpio	Water	Fruitful	3rd
14 Wed.	Scorpio	Water	Fruitful	4th 10:23 pm
15 Thu. 5:02 am	Sagittarius	Fire	Barren	4th
16 Fri.	Sagittarius	Fire	Barren	4th
17 Sat. 3:59 pm	Capricorn	Earth	Semi-fruit	4th
18 Sun.	Capricorn	Earth	Semi-fruit	4th
19 Mon.	Capricorn	Earth	Semi-fruit	4th
20 Tue. 4:53 am	Aquarius	Air	Barren	4th
21 Wed.	Aquarius	Air	Barren	4th
22 Thu. 5:45 pm	Pisces	Water	Fruitful	4th
23 Fri.	Pisces	Water	Fruitful	1st 3:21 am
24 Sat.	Pisces	Water	Fruitful	1st
25 Sun. 5:20 am	Aries	Fire	Barren	1st
26 Mon.	Aries	Fire	Barren	1st
27 Tue. 3:06 pm	Taurus	Earth	Semi-fruit	1st
28 Wed.	Taurus	Earth	Semi-fruit	1st

March Moon Table

Date	Sign	Element	Nature	Phase
1 Thu. 10:36 pm	Gemini	Air	Barren	1st
2 Fri.	Gemini	Air	Barren	2nd 9:03 pm
3 Sat.	Gemini	Air	Barren	2nd
4 Sun. 3:24 am	Cancer	Water	Fruitful	2nd
5 Mon.	Cancer	Water	Fruitful	2nd
6 Tue. 5:30 am	Leo	Fire	Barren	2nd
7 Wed.	Leo	Fire	Barren	2nd
8 Thu. 5:44 am	Virgo	Earth	Barren	2nd
9 Fri.	Virgo	Earth	Barren	3rd 12:23 pm
10 Sat. 5:47 am	Libra	Air	Semi-fruit	3rd
11 Sun.	Libra	Air	Semi-fruit	3rd
12 Mon. 7:43 am	Scorpio	Water	Fruitful	3rd
13 Tue.	Scorpio	Water	Fruitful	3rd
14 Wed. 1:17 pm	Sagittarius	Fire	Barren	3rd
15 Thu.	Sagittarius	Fire	Barren	3rd
16 Fri. 11:02 pm	Capricorn	Earth	Semi-fruit	4th 3:45 pm
17 Sat.	Capricorn	Earth	Semi-fruit	4th
18 Sun.	Capricorn	Earth	Semi-fruit	4th
19 Mon. 11:36 am	Aquarius	Air	Barren	4th
20 Tue.	Aquarius	Air	Barren	4th
21 Wed.	Aquarius	Air	Barren	4th
22 Thu. 12:28 am	Pisces	Water	Fruitful	4th
23 Fri.	Pisces	Water	Fruitful	4th
24 Sat. 11:43 am	Aries	Fire	Barren	1st 8:21 pm
25 Sun.	Aries	Fire	Barren	1st
26 Mon. 8:50 pm	Taurus	Earth	Semi-fruit	1st
27 Tue.	Taurus	Earth	Semi-fruit	1st
28 Wed.	Taurus	Earth	Semi-fruit	1st
29 Thu. 4:01 am	Gemini	Air	Barren	1st
30 Fri.	Gemini	Air	Barren	1st
31 Sat. 9:23 am	Cancer	Water	Fruitful	1st

April Moon Table

Date	Sign	Element	Nature	Phase
1 Sun.	Can.	Water	Fruitful	2nd 5:49 am
2 Mon. 12:54 pm	Leo	Fire	Barren	2nd
3 Tue.	Leo	Fire	Barren	2nd
4 Wed. 2:46 pm	Virgo	Earth	Barren	2nd
5 Thu.	Virgo	Earth	Barren	2nd
6 Fri. 3:57 pm	Libra	Air	Semi-fruit	2nd
7 Sat.	Libra	Air	Semi-fruit	3rd 10:22 pm
8 Sun. 6:01 pm	Scorpio	Water	Fruitful	3rd
9 Mon.	Scorpio	Water	Fruitful	3rd
10 Tue. 10:47 pm	Sagittarius	Fire	Barren	3rd
11 Wed.	Sagittarius	Fire	Barren	3rd
12 Thu.	Sagittarius	Fire	Barren	3rd
13 Fri. 7:21 am	Capricorn	Earth	Semi-fruit	3rd
14 Sat.	Capricorn	Earth	Semi-fruit	3rd
15 Sun. 7:11 pm	Aquarius	Air	Barren	4th 10:31 am
16 Mon.	Aquarius	Air	Barren	4th
17 Tue.	Aquarius	Air	Barren	4th
18 Wed. 8:00 am	Pisces	Water	Fruitful	4th
19 Thu.	Pisces	Water	Fruitful	4th
20 Fri. 7:18 pm	Aries	Fire	Barren	4th
21 Sat.	Aries	Fire	Barren	4th
22 Sun.	Aries	Fire	Barren	4th
23 Mon. 3:56 am	Taurus	Earth	Semi-fruit	1st 10:26 am
24 Tue.	Taurus	Earth	Semi-fruit	1st
25 Wed. 10:11 am	Gemini	Air	Barren	1st
26 Thu.	Gemini	Air	Barren	1st
27 Fri. 2:49 pm	CAN	Water	Fruitful	1st
28 Sat.	CAN	Water	Fruitful	1st
29 Sun. 6:25 pm	Leo	Fire	Barren	1st
30 Mon.	Leo	Fire	Barren	2nd 12:08 pm

May Moon Table

Date	Sign	Element	Nature	Phase
1 Tue. 9:16 pm	Virgo	Earth	Barren	2nd
2 Wed.	Virgo	Earth	Barren	2nd
3 Thu. 11:50 pm	Libra	Air	Semi-fruit	2nd
4 Fri.	Libra	Air	Semi-fruit	2nd
5 Sat.	Libra	Air	Semi-fruit	2nd
6 Sun. 3:00 am	Scorpio	Water	Fruitful	2nd
7 Mon.	Scorpio	Water	Fruitful	3rd 8:53 am
8 Tue. 8:05 am	Sagittarius	Fire	Barren	3rd
9 Wed.	Sagittarius	Fire	Barren	3rd
10 Thu. 4:10 pm	Capricorn	Earth	Semi-fruit	3rd
11 Fri.	Capricorn	Earth	Semi-fruit	3rd
12 Sat.	Capricorn	Earth	Semi-fruit	3rd
13 Sun. 3:20 am	Aquarius	Air	Barren	3rd
14 Mon.	Aquarius	Air	Barren	3rd
15 Tue. 4:01 pm	Pisces	Water	Fruitful	4th 5:11 am
16 Wed.	Pisces	Water	Fruitful	4th
17 Thu.	Pisces	Water	Fruitful	4th
18 Fri. 3:41 am	Aries	Fire	Barren	4th
19 Sat.	Aries	Fire	Barren	4th
20 Sun. 12:29 pm	Taurus	Earth	Semi-fruit	4th
21 Mon.	Taurus	Earth	Semi-fruit	4th
22 Tue. 6:12 pm	Gemini	Air	Barren	1st 9:46 pm
23 Wed.	Gemini	Air	Barren	1st
24 Thu. 9:42 pm	Cancer	Water	Fruitful	1st
25 Fri.	Cancer	Water	Fruitful	1st
26 Sat.	Cancer	Water	Fruitful	1st
27 Sun. 12:12 am	Leo	Fire	Barren	1st
28 Mon.	Leo	Fire	Barren	1st
29 Tue. 2:38 am	Virgo	Earth	Barren	2nd 5:09 pm
30 Wed.	Virgo	Earth	Barren	2nd
31 Thu. 5:41 am	Libra	Air	Semi-fruit	2nd

June Moon Table

Date	Sign	Element	Nature	Phase
1 Fri.	Libra	Air	Semi-fruit	2nd
2 Sat. 9:56 am	Scorpio	Water	Fruitful	2nd
3 Sun.	Scorpio	Water	Fruitful	2nd
4 Mon. 3:58 pm	Sagittarius	Fire	Barren	2nd
5 Tue.	Sagittarius	Fire	Barren	3rd 8:39 pm
6 Wed.	Sagittarius	Fire	Barren	3rd
7 Thu. 12:23 am	Capricorn	Earth	Semi-fruit	3rd
8 Fri.	Capricorn	Earth	Semi-fruit	3rd
9 Sat. 11:20 am	Aquarius	Air	Barren	3rd
10 Sun.	Aquarius	Air	Barren	3rd
11 Mon. 11:53 pm	Pisces	Water	Fruitful	3rd
12 Tue.	Pisces	Water	Fruitful	3rd
13 Wed.	Pisces	Water	Fruitful	4th 10:28 pm
14 Thu. 12:03 pm	Aries	Fire	Barren	4th
15 Fri.	Aries	Fire	Barren	4th
16 Sat. 9:39 pm	Taurus	Earth	Semi-fruit	4th
17 Sun.	Taurus	Earth	Semi-fruit	4th
18 Mon.	Taurus	Earth	Semi-fruit	4th
19 Tue. 3:42 am	Gemini	Air	Barren	4th
20 Wed.	Gemini	Air	Barren	4th
21 Thu. 6:40 am	Cancer	Water	Fruitful	1st 6:58 am
22 Fri.	Cancer	Water	Fruitful	1st
23 Sat. 7:55 am	Leo	Fire	Barren	1st
24 Sun.	Leo	Fire	Barren	1st
25 Mon. 8:57 am	Virgo	Earth	Barren	1st
26 Tue.	Virgo	Earth	Barren	1st
27 Wed. 11:11 am	Libra	Air	Semi-fruit	2nd 10:19 pm
28 Thu.	Libra	Air	Semi-fruit	2nd
29 Fri. 3:28 pm	Scorpio	Water	Fruitful	2nd
30 Sat.	Scorpio	Water	Fruitful	2nd

July Moon Table

Date	Sign	Element	Nature	Phase
1 Sun. 10:13 pm	Sagittarius	Fire	Barren	2nd
2 Mon.	Sagittarius	Fire	Barren	2nd
3 Tue.	Sagittarius	Fire	Barren	2nd
4 Wed. 7:21 am	Capricorn	Earth	Semi-fruit	2nd
5 Thu.	Capricorn	Earth	Semi-fruit	3rd 10:04 am
6 Fri. 6:33 pm	Aquarius	Air	Barren	3rd
7 Sat.	Aquarius	Air	Barren	3rd
8 Sun.	Aquarius	Air	Barren	3rd
9 Mon. 7:05 am	Pisces	Water	Fruitful	3rd
10 Tue.	Pisces	Water	Fruitful	3rd
11 Wed. 7:36 pm	Aries	Fire	Barren	3rd
12 Thu.	Aries	Fire	Barren	3rd
13 Fri.	Aries	Fire	Barren	4th 1:45 pm
14 Sat. 6:13 am	Taurus	Earth	Semi-fruit	4th
15 Sun.	Taurus	Earth	Semi-fruit	4th
16 Mon. 1:26 pm	Gemini	Air	Barren	4th
17 Tue.	Gemini	Air	Barren	4th
18 Wed. 4:56 pm	Cancer	Water	Fruitful	4th
19 Thu.	Cancer	Water	Fruitful	4th
20 Fri. 5:43 pm	Leo	Fire	Barren	1st 2:44 pm
21 Sat.	Leo	Fire	Barren	1st
22 Sun. 5:29 pm	Virgo	Earth	Barren	1st
23 Mon.	Virgo	Earth	Barren	1st
24 Tue. 6:08 pm	Libra	Air	Semi-fruit	1st
25 Wed.	Libra	Air	Semi-fruit	1st
26 Thu. 9:17 pm	Scorpio	Water	Fruitful	1st
27 Fri.	Scorpio	Water	Fruitful	2nd 5:08 am
28 Sat.	Scorpio	Water	Fruitful	2nd
29 Sun. 3:44 am	Sagittarius	Fire	Barren	2nd
30 Mon.	Sagittarius	Fire	Barren	2nd
31 Tue. 1:16 pm	Capricorn	Earth	Semi-fruit	2nd

August Moon Table

Date	Sign	Element	Nature	Phase
1 Wed.	Capricorn	Earth	Semi-fruit	2nd
2 Thu.	Capricorn	Earth	Semi-fruit	2nd
3 Fri. 12:53 am	Aquarius	Air	Barren	2nd
4 Sat.	Aquarius	Air	Barren	3rd 12:56 am
5 Sun. 1:30 pm	Pisces	Water	Fruitful	3rd
6 Mon.	Pisces	Water	Fruitful	3rd
7 Tue.	Pisces	Water	Fruitful	3rd
8 Wed. 2:05 am	Aries	Fire	Barren	3rd
9 Thu.	Aries	Fire	Barren	3rd
10 Fri. 1:23 pm	Taurus	Earth	Semi-fruit	3rd
11 Sat.	Taurus	Earth	Semi-fruit	3rd
12 Sun. 9:59 pm	Gemini	Air	Barren	4th 2:53 am
13 Mon.	Gemini	Air	Barren	4th
14 Tue.	Gemini	Air	Barren	4th
15 Wed. 2:55 am	Cancer	Water	Fruitful	4th
16 Thu.	Cancer	Water	Fruitful	4th
17 Fri. 4:25 am	Leo	Fire	Barren	4th
18 Sat.	Leo	Fire	Barren	1st 9:55 pm
19 Sun. 3:53 am	Virgo	Earth	Barren	1st
20 Mon.	Virgo	Earth	Barren	1st
21 Tue. 3:19 am	Libra	Air	Semi-fruit	1st
22 Wed.	Libra	Air	Semi-fruit	1st
23 Thu. 4:50 am	Scorpio	Water	Fruitful	1st
24 Fri.	Scorpio	Water	Fruitful	1st
25 Sat. 9:59 am	Sagittarius	Fire	Barren	2nd 2:55 pm
26 Sun.	Sagittarius	Fire	Barren	2nd
27 Mon. 7:02 pm	Capricorn	Earth	Semi-fruit	2nd
28 Tue.	Capricorn	Earth	Semi-fruit	2nd
29 Wed.	Capricorn	Earth	Semi-fruit	2nd
30 Thu. 6:47 am	Aquarius	Air	Barren	2nd
31 Fri.	Aquarius	Air	Barren	2nd

September Moon Table

Date	Sign	Element	Nature	Phase
1 Sat. 7:32 pm	Pisces	Water	Fruitful	2nd
2 Sun.	Pisces	Water	Fruitful	3rd 4:43 pm
3 Mon.	Pisces	Water	Fruitful	3rd
4 Tue. 7:58 am	Aries	Fire	Barren	3rd
5 Wed.	Aries	Fire	Barren	3rd
6 Thu. 7:18 pm	Taurus	Earth	Semi-fruit	3rd
7 Fri.	Taurus	Earth	Semi-fruit	3rd
8 Sat.	Taurus	Earth	Semi-fruit	3rd
9 Sun. 4:41 am	Gemini	Air	Barren	3rd
10 Mon.	Gemini	Air	Barren	4th 1:59 pm
11 Tue. 11:09 am	Cancer	Water	Fruitful	4th
12 Wed.	Cancer	Water	Fruitful	4th
13 Thu. 2:16 pm	Leo	Fire	Barren	4th
14 Fri.	Leo	Fire	Barren	4th
15 Sat. 2:39 pm	Virgo	Earth	Barren	4th
16 Sun.	Virgo	Earth	Barren	4th
17 Mon. 2:00 pm	Libra	Air	Semi-fruit	1st 5:27 am
18 Tue.	Libra	Air	Semi-fruit	1st
19 Wed. 2:27 pm	Scorpio	Water	Fruitful	1st
20 Thu.	Scorpio	Water	Fruitful	1st
21 Fri. 6:02 pm	Sagittarius	Fire	Barren	1st
22 Sat.	Sagittarius	Fire	Barren	1st
23 Sun.	Sagittarius	Fire	Barren	1st
24 Mon. 1:48 am	Capricorn	Earth	Semi-fruit	2nd 4:31 am
25 Tue.	Capricorn	Earth	Semi-fruit	2nd
26 Wed. 1:05 pm	Aquarius	Air	Barren	2nd
27 Thu.	Aquarius	Air	Barren	2nd
28 Fri.	Aquarius	Air	Barren	2nd
29 Sat. 1:50 am	Pisces	Water	Fruitful	2nd
30 Sun.	Pisces	Water	Fruitful	2nd

October Moon Table

Date	Sign	Element	Nature	Phase
1 Mon. 2:08 pm	Aries	Fire	Barren	2nd
2 Tue.	Aries	Fire	Barren	3rd 8:49 am
3 Wed.	Aries	Fire	Barren	3rd
4 Thu. 1:01 am	Taurus	Earth	Semi-fruit	3rd
5 Fri.	Taurus	Earth	Semi-fruit	3rd
6 Sat. 10:12 am	Gemini	Air	Barren	3rd
7 Sun.	Gemini	Air	Barren	3rd
8 Mon. 5:19 pm	Cancer	Water	Fruitful	3rd
9 Tue.	Cancer	Water	Fruitful	4th 11:20 pm
10 Wed. 9:54 pm	Leo	Fire	Barren	4th
11 Thu.	Leo	Fire	Barren	4th
12 Fri. 11:58 pm	Virgo	Earth	Barren	4th
13 Sat.	Virgo	Earth	Barren	4th
14 Sun.	Virgo	Earth	Barren	4th
15 Mon. 12:26 am	Libra	Air	Semi-fruit	4th
16 Tue.	Libra	Air	Semi-fruit	1st 2:23 pm
17 Wed. 1:03 am	Scorpio	Water	Fruitful	1st
18 Thu.	Scorpio	Water	Fruitful	1st
19 Fri. 3:47 am	Sagittarius	Fire	Barren	1st
20 Sat.	Sagittarius	Fire	Barren	1st
21 Sun. 10:11 am	Capricorn	Earth	Semi-fruit	1st
22 Mon.	Capricorn	Earth	Semi-fruit	1st
23 Tue. 8:26 pm	Aquarius	Air	Barren	2nd 9:58 pm
24 Wed.	Aquarius	Air	Barren	2nd
25 Thu.	Aquarius	Air	Barren	2nd
26 Fri. 8:56 am	Pisces	Water	Fruitful	2nd
27 Sat.	Pisces	Water	Fruitful	2nd
28 Sun. 9:15 pm	Aries	Fire	Barren	2nd
29 Mon.	Aries	Fire	Barren	2nd
30 Tue.	Aries	Fire	Barren	2nd
31 Wed. 7:48 am	Taurus	Earth	Semi-fruit	2nd

November Moon Table

Date	Sign	Element	Nature	Phase
1 Thu.	Taurus	Earth	Semi-fruit	3rd 12:41 am
2 Fri. 4:12 pm	Gemini	Air	Barren	3rd
3 Sat.	Gemini	Air	Barren	3rd
4 Sun. 10:44 pm	Cancer	Water	Fruitful	3rd
5 Mon.	Cancer	Water	Fruitful	3rd
6 Tue.	Cancer	Water	Fruitful	3rd
7 Wed. 3:34 am	Leo	Fire	Barren	3rd
8 Thu.	Leo	Fire	Barren	4th 7:21 am
9 Fri. 6:49 am	Virgo	Earth	Barren	4th
10 Sat.	Virgo	Earth	Barren	4th
11 Sun. 8:53 am	Libra	Air	Semi-fruit	4th
12 Mon.	Libra	Air	Semi-fruit	4th
13 Tue. 10:44 am	Scorpio	Water	Fruitful	4th
14 Wed.	Scorpio	Water	Fruitful	4th
15 Thu. 1:51 pm	Sagittarius	Fire	Barren	1st 1:40 am
16 Fri.	Sagittarius	Fire	Barren	1st
17 Sat. 7:40 pm	Capricorn	Earth	Semi-fruit	1st
18 Sun.	Capricorn	Earth	Semi-fruit	1st
19 Mon.	Capricorn	Earth	Semi-fruit	1st
20 Tue. 4:55 am	Aquarius	Air	Barren	1st
21 Wed.	Aquarius	Air	Barren	1st
22 Thu. 4:52 pm	Pisces	Water	Fruitful	2nd 6:21 pm
23 Fri.	Pisces	Water	Fruitful	2nd
24 Sat.	Pisces	Water	Fruitful	2nd
25 Sun. 5:21 am	Aries	Fire	Barren	2nd
26 Mon.	Aries	Fire	Barren	2nd
27 Tue. 4:06 pm	Taurus	Earth	Semi-fruit	2nd
28 Wed.	Taurus	Earth	Semi-fruit	2nd
29 Thu.	Taurus	Earth	Semi-fruit	2nd
30 Fri. 12:04 am	Gemini	Air	Barren	3rd 3:49 pm

December Moon Table

Date	Sign	Element	Nature	Phase
1 Sat.	Gemini	Air	Barren	3rd
2 Sun. 5:30 am	Cancer	Water	Fruitful	3rd
3 Mon.	Cancer	Water	Fruitful	3rd
4 Tue. 9:15 am	Leo	Fire	Barren	3rd
5 Wed.	Leo	Fire	Barren	3rd
6 Thu. 12:11 pm	Virgo	Earth	Barren	3rd
7 Fri.	Virgo	Earth	Barren	4th 2:52 pm
8 Sat. 2:57 pm	Libra	Air	Semi-fruit	4th
9 Sun.	Libra	Air	Semi-fruit	4th
10 Mon. 6:09 pm	Scorpio	Water	Fruitful	4th
11 Tue.	Scorpio	Water	Fruitful	4th
12 Wed. 10:30 pm	Sagittarius	Fire	Barren	4th
13 Thu.	Sagittarius	Fire	Barren	4th
14 Fri.	Sagittarius	Fire	Barren	1st 3:47 pm
15 Sat. 4:48 am	Capricorn	Earth	Semi-fruit	1st
16 Sun.	Capricorn	Earth	Semi-fruit	1st
17 Mon. 1:43 pm	Aquarius	Air	Barren	1st
18 Tue.	Aquarius	Air	Barren	1st
19 Wed.	Aquarius	Air	Barren	1st
20 Thu. 1:09 am	Pisces	Water	Fruitful	1st
21 Fri.	Pisces	Water	Fruitful	1st
22 Sat. 1:45 pm	Aries	Fire	Barren	2nd 3:56 pm
23 Sun.	Aries	Fire	Barren	2nd
24 Mon.	Aries	Fire	Barren	2nd
25 Tue. 1:12 am	Taurus	Earth	Semi-fruit	2nd
26 Wed.	Taurus	Earth	Semi-fruit	2nd
27 Thu. 9:39 am	Gemini	Air	Barren	2nd
28 Fri.	Gemini	Air	Barren	2nd
29 Sat. 2:40 pm	Cancer	Water	Fruitful	2nd
30 Sun.	Cancer	Water	Fruitful	3rd 5:40 am
31 Mon. 5:09 pm	Leo	Fire	Barren	3rd

About the Authors

BERNYCE BARLOW is author of Llewellyn's *Sacred Sites of the West* and has been a contributer to the Llewellyn almanacs since 1995. She is a researcher, speaker, and leads sacred site seminars throughout the United States. She is best known for her magical tools of enlightment that come from the *Acme* toy company, and she swears that her cartoon totems are real!

ELIZABETH BARRETTE is a regular contributor to *SageWoman*, *PanGaia*, *Circle Network News*, *PagaNet News*, and *Moonbeams Journal*. Much of her involvement with the wider Pagan community takes place online, where she has helped build networking resources such as the Pagan Leaders mailing list. Visit her website at http://www.worthlink. net/~ysabet/index.html.

GERINA DUNWICH is a high priestess of the Old Religion, a professional astrologer, cat lover, Tarot reader, and the author of numerous books. The founder of The Pagan Poets Society, The Wheel of Wisdom School, and Golden Isis Press, she currently resides in California with her Gemini lover and a black cat named Salem. Her website is at www.geocities.com/Area51/Atlantis/1978.

MARGUERITE ELSBETH (also known as Senihele and Sparrow Hawk) is an hereditary Sicilian strega and part Lenni Lenape (Delaware) Indian. She is a professional tarot reader, astrologer, and practitioner of Nativism (American Indian healing). She has published numerous articles in Llewellyn's annuals, is the author of the Llewellyn books *Crystal Medicine*, *The Grail Castle: Male Myths and Mysteries in the Celtic Tradition* and *The Silver Wheel: Women's Myths and Mysteries in the Celtic Tradition* (both with Kenneth Johnson). She currently resides in the Southwest.

JUDY GRIFFIN, PH.D. is an international lecturer, counselor, and author. She has researched indigenous cultures for twenty years and is an authority on medicinal herbs, aromatherapy, skincare, flower essences, and gardening. She has written *Mother Nature's Herbal* (Llewellyn, 1997), a 400-page herbal recently featured on PBS. Judy is presently leading an aromatherapy study with bone marrow and stem cell transplant patients at the Baylor Medical Healing Environment Center. She also privately consults as a nutritionist and herbalist.

DEBORAH HARDING has been studying herbs for over twenty years, and she plans to continue studying them for the rest of her life. She is the author of Llewellyn's *Green Guide to Herb Gardening*, and she is a musician who performs with her husband and two daughters at Renaissance Fairs. She is also an artist specializing in American folk, fantasy, and Native American art.

EILEEN HOLLAND is a witch who began researching for her personal grimoire while living in Egypt. She is the author of *The Wicca Handbook* (Weiser, 2000), and webmaster of Open, Sesame (www.open-sesame.com), a popular Wiccan website that has sections on herb and tree lore.

ELLEN EVERT HOPMAN is the author of *Tree Medicine, Tree Magic* (Phoenix, 1991), *A Druid's Herbal for the Sacred Earth Year* (Destiny, 1995), *People of the Earth: New Pagans Speak Out* (Destiny, 1996), as well as the videos *Gifts from the Healing Earth* and *Pagans* (EFP Services). She can be contacted through her website at: http://www.neopagan.net/WillowsGrove/Index.html.

LIZ JOHNSON provided supplementary herbal proofreading for this almanac. She is co-owner of Firewind Herbal Products, which makes quality incense, candles, soap, jewelry, and other products for Wiccans and magical people. To request a catalog call 612/543-9065 or find them on the Internet at www.firewindhp.com.

PENNY KELLY has earned a degree in naturopathic medicine and is working toward a Ph.D. in nutition. She is the author of the book *The Elves of Lily Hill Farm*.

GRETCHEN LAWLOR has been an astrologer and a naturopathic medical practitioner for more than 25 years. She incorporates homeopathic flower remedies, herbs, and supplements into her practice, and she teaches natural approaches to health problems to hospital groups and alternative medical practitioners. She has been a contributor to Llewellyn's annuals for many years and can be reached through her website at www.glawlor.hypermart.com.

CAROLINE MOSS holds workshops and lectures in Cheshire, England to teach about growing and using herbs, and she designs herb gardens. She shares her home with a husband, two children, and a menagerie of pets, including hens, ponies, and sheep.

LEEDA ALLEYN PACOTTI is a naturopathic physician, specializing in health crises involving subtle bodies. She uses ancient traditions and herbal and flower remedies in her practice, counsels in health astrology, and pursues ground-breaking research in dream language to dignose health states.

ROSLYN REID is a Discordian Druid and a member of the Richard P. Feynman Memorial Cabal. She lives on a fruit farm and raises Pyrenees dogs. She teaches yoga and tarot, and is a regular contributor of art and articles to Llewellyn, as well as to Pagan oriented publications such as *SageWoman* and *Dalriada*. She has also published pieces in consumer magazines such as *Tightwad Living* and *Thrifty Times*, and was a contributor Susun Weed's book, *Breast Cancer? Breast Health! The Wise Woman Way* (Ash Tree, 1996).

SILVER SAGE, an elder in the Celtic tradition, is a wife, mother, and grandmother, and a dedicated student of the herb world for over twenty years. Living in the Southern California mountains, with her husband of thirty years, Sage runs Dances with Herbs, a retail herb shop, where she strives to provide information everyone on the human and magical use of herbs. She has also designed and written her own web page: "Silver Sage: The Outrageous Herb Lady," located at: www.herbanspice.com/silversage/index.html

K.D. SPITZER has loved herbs all her life. In the years before they became readily available, she wildcrafted plants from the woods and abandoned cellar holes and relied on her French mother-in-law to send seeds from Europe. She is a master weaver, and one corner of her herb garden is devoted to dye herbs. She teaches in New Hampshire, where she also reads tarot.

CARLY WALL, C.A. is the author of *Flower Secrets Revealed: Using flowers to Heal, Beautify and Energize Your Life!* (ARE Press, 1993), *Naturally Healing Herbs* (Sterling, 1996), and *The Little Encyclopedia of Olde Thyme Home Remedies* (Sterling, 2000). A regular contributor to Llewellyn's annuals for the last seven years, she holds a certificate in aromatherapy and lives on a farm with her husband, Ron and cat, Missy.

(Editor's Note: The contents of this book are not meant to diagnose, treat, prescribe, or substitute for consultation with a licensed heath care professional. Herbs, whether used internally or externally, should be introduced in small amounts to allow the body to adjust and to detect possible allergies. Llewellyn Worldwide does not participate in, endorse, or have any authority or responsibility concerning private business transactions between its authors and the public.)